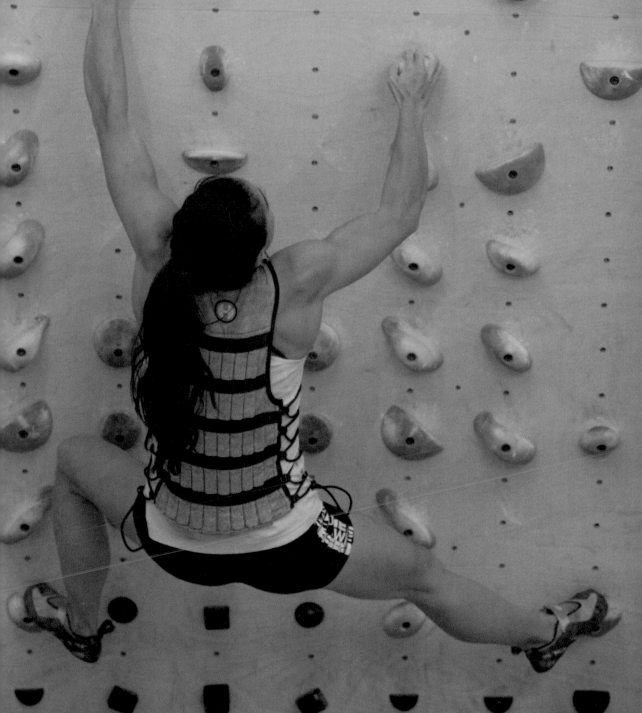

Climbing

Climb to Fitness

Special thanks to photographer Kris Ugarriza (Red Wave Pictures), photo assistant Molly Stern, fitness models Nina Williams and James Lucas, research assistant Zoe Gates, and EVO Rock + Fitness in Louisville, Colorado.

FALCONGUIDES®

An imprint of The Rowman & Littlefield Publishing Group, Inc.
4501 Forbes Blvd., Ste. 200
Lanham, MD 20706

Falcon and FalconGuides are registered trademarks, and Make Adventure Your Story is a trademark of The Rowman & Littlefield Publishing Group, Inc.

Distributed by NATIONAL BOOK NETWORK
Copyright © 2018 Climbing magazine, a division of Active Interest Media

Photos by Kris Ugarriza (Red Wave Pictures)

Text adjusted from original text by the following contributors: Steve Bechtel, Alex Biale, Brendan Blanchard, Kevin Corrigan, Shannon Davis, Dan Dewell, Julie Ellison, Robyn Erbesfield-Raboutou, Mic Fairchild, Amanda Fox, Eric Hörst, James Lucas, Dougald MacDonald, Dave MacLeod, Theresa Maruyama, Stacy McCooey, Caroline Meleedy, Hailey Moore, Kris Peters, Rob Pizem, Andy Raether, Alli Rainey, Max Ritter, Adam Scheer, Lizzy Scully, Dave Sheldon, Justen Sjong, Abbey Smith, Andrew Tower, Dave Wahl, Kyle Ward, JP Whitehead, and Heidi Wirtz.

British Library Cataloguing in Publication Information available

Library of Congress Cataloging-in-Publication Data available

ISBN 978-1-4930-3054-5
ISBN 978-1-4930-3065-1 (e-book)

♾™ The paper used in this publication meets the minimum requirements of American National Standard for Information Sciences—Permanence of Paper for Printed Library Materials, ANSI/NISO Z39.48-1992.

Printed in the United States of America

Warning: Climbing is a dangerous sport. You can be seriously injured or die. Read the following before you use this book.
This is an instruction book about rock climbing, a sport that is inherently dangerous. Do not depend solely on information from this book for your personal safety. Your climbing safety depends on your own judgment based on competent instruction, experience, and a realistic assessment of your climbing ability.

The training advice given in this book is based on the author's opinions. Consult your physician before engaging in any part of the training program described by the author.

There are no warranties, either expressed or implied, that this instruction book contains accurate and reliable information. There are no warranties as to fitness for a particular purpose or that this book is merchantable. Your use of this book indicates your assumption of the risk of death or serious injury as a result of climbing's risks and is an acknowledgment of your own sole responsibility for your safety in climbing or in training for climbing.

Rowman & Littlefield and the author assume no liability for accidents happening to, or injuries sustained by, readers who engage in the activities described in this book.

Climbing

Climb to Fitness

The Ultimate Guide
to Customizing a
Powerful Workout
on the Wall

Julie Ellison

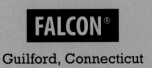

Guilford, Connecticut

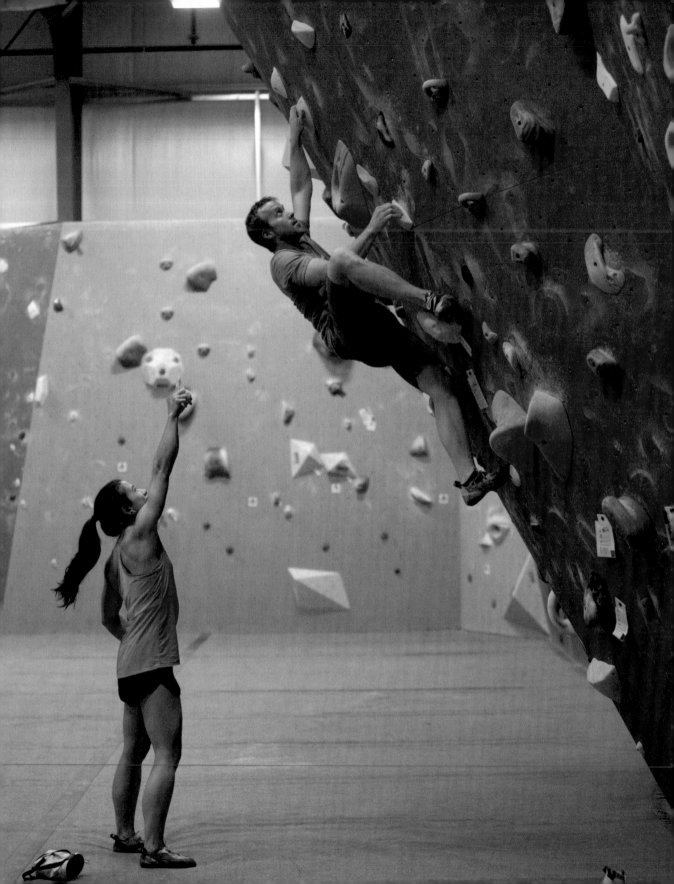

Contents

Introduction 7

Chapter 1: Basics of Gym Climbing — 13

Chapter 2: Strength — 35

Chapter 3: Endurance — 69

Chapter 4: Climbing Supplements — 99

Chapter 5: Off-the-Wall Fitness — 135

Chapter 6: Climb a Grade Harder — 195

Index of Exercises: Quick Reference **242**

Glossary of Terms **249**

About the Author **256**

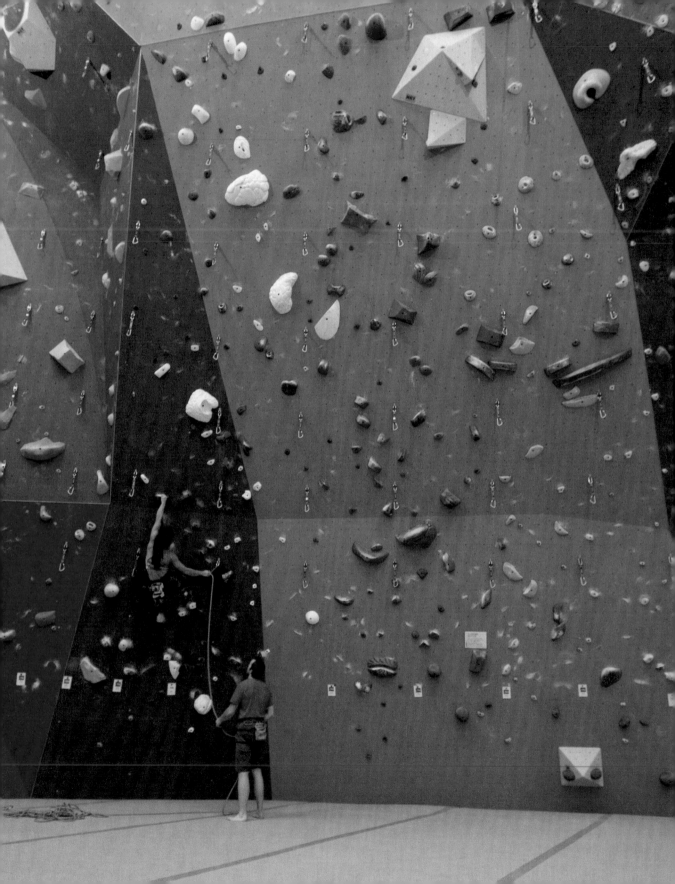

INTRODUCTION

AS THE NUMBER OF CLIMBING GYMS across the country continues to grow, people have caught on to a secret that longtime climbers have always known: climbing is *fun*. More interesting than running on a treadmill or lifting weights over and over, climbing offers a unique way to get fit. Depending on the style you choose—longer routes on a rope or ropeless climbing on shorter boulders—climbing offers a nice combination of aerobic and anaerobic exercise. Each time you pull onto the wall, you're guaranteed to use almost every muscle in your body, from your feet, legs, and hips to your core, shoulders, and arms. This is why seasoned climbers have muscular physiques, with well-developed deltoids, latissimus dorsi (lats), biceps, and forearms. Those muscles stand out because the mix of anaerobic and aerobic demands is a perfect recipe for burning fat.

Climbing even utilizes our most important muscle: the brain. Tricky hand and foot sequences demand strategy, thoughtful movement, and body awareness, and technique is just as important as physical strength. Because each climb is given a number grade, it's fun to track your progress as you climb more. There's always something harder to climb, so it's easy to stay motivated and keep improving.

Another incentive is the social aspect of climbing. With roped climbing, you must have a partner to belay you, and when bouldering, you spend a lot of time standing on the ground discussing beta and chatting with other climbers. There are usually couches or tables in gyms, where climbers can just hang out together, and when you develop a network of climber friends, there's a good chance that you'll get daily invites to the gym. What other type of exercise has accountability like that?

Then there's the climbing gym itself. Because many gyms have been built within the last ten years, they're shiny and new, with modern equipment, colorful aesthetics, and environmentally friendly design elements, like solar power and low-energy consumption. Many of them have fitness classes, spinning classes, yoga, personal trainers, climbing coaches, weight rooms, Wi-Fi, and showers. Some of the newest gyms even have juice bars, retail stores, and coworking spaces. Climbing gyms are fun places to spend time, and the more you're there, the fitter you'll get.

Chances are, even if you've just started climbing, you're already totally addicted and just want to climb. In the beginning, you'll see drastic improvements day after day, and that might be enough to keep you coming back for more. Eventually you'll

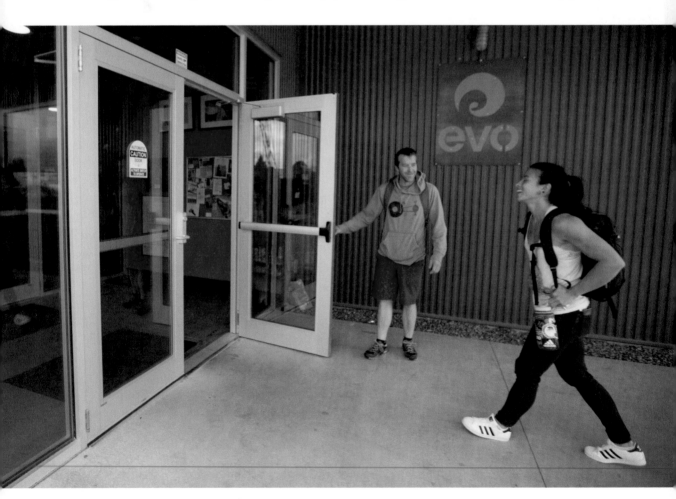

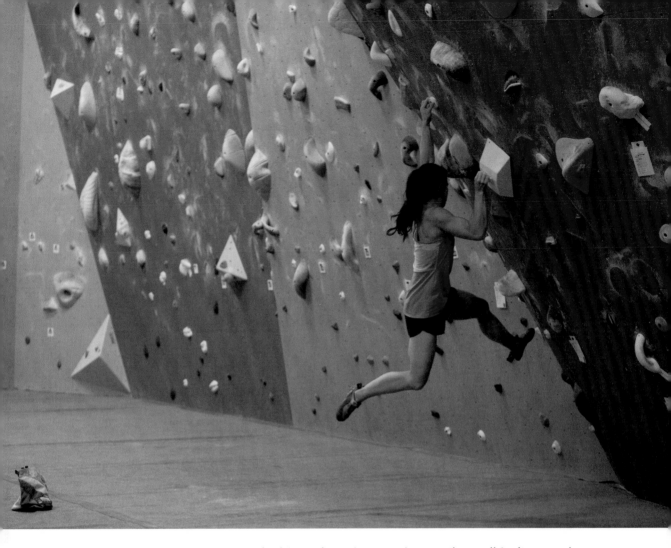

plateau, or hit a point in your climbing where just getting on the wall isn't enough to get better. That's where this book comes in. Whether you're new to the gym and your goal is general fitness or you're an experienced climber whose goal is to climb a certain grade, *Climb to Fitness* will help you structure your time at the gym so you reach your personal goal, even if that goal is just to have fun.

How to Use This Book

Climb to Fitness is organized into six main chapters. Each chapter has up to ten "workouts" geared toward specific fitness goals: strength, endurance, climbing supplements, and off-the-wall fitness, which means exercise for your whole body. Many of the workouts are meant to be one-offs, so if you're looking for something to do on any single session at the gym, there are plenty of options to choose from.

A Note about Autobelays and Partners

Many gyms have autobelays, devices that take in slack as you move up so you can climb roped routes without a partner. All you have to do is clip in and climb up, then when you reach the top of the wall or take a fall, the autobelay device catches you and lowers you slowly. Most of the roped climbing workouts in this book require a partner, but keep in mind that an autobelay can be your partner. If there's a particular workout you'd like to do, you can customize it to be done with the autobelay. Make sure to get specific instruction on how to use the autobelay from your local gym.

Think of it as an a la carte menu—mix-and-match however you'd like to get a good workout. You can also use these individual workouts to build a long-term program, where you follow a set schedule of doing certain workouts on certain days. If you'd rather not design a program like that yourself, we've also included a few long-term programs where everything is already laid out for you day-by-day, week-by-week, and month-by-month. You'll find those in the gray pages near the end of each chapter. Try out all of these approaches—single workouts, mix-and-match, structured long-term training—to find what works best for you, your psych, and your schedule. Don't do more than one long-term program from Chapters 2 and 3 at once; that's too much training. You can, however, add the long-term programs in Chapter 4 to one-off workouts. Because we know you might be limited by constraints of daily life—time, partner availability, energy—we've included a handy Index of Exercises in the back of the book (page 242) where you'll find each workout organized by factors that include how long the workout will take, intensity level, type of climbing, partner requirement, and whether it's a long-term program or a one-off workout. The index is a good starting point if you don't know which type of fitness you want to train for on a particular day. Climbing is an activity filled with specific jargon, so if there's a word or phrase that you don't understand, check the glossary that starts on page 249.

If you want to pick a workout based on a specific goal, then use the following guidelines:

▶ Strength focuses on pure power and the ability to perform certain movements.

- ▶ Endurance will improve your ability to perform those certain movements over a long period of time.

- ▶ The Climbing Supplements chapter shows you how to use specialized tools (hangboard, campus board, system board) for training climbing.

- ▶ Off-the-Wall Fitness heads to the weight room and yoga studio. This chapter covers full-body fitness, which will also make you a stronger climber and, more importantly, will teach you injury-prevention exercises, a crucial aspect of training.

- ▶ The last chapter, Climb a Grade Harder, combines all the fitness goals into one nine-week program that will help you, well, climb a grade harder. This training regimen incorporates aspects of every other chapter in a thoughtful plan that will make you a stronger climber. If you like following a long-term plan instead of piecing together your own training, consider this chapter.

If you're completely new to climbing, or new to training for climbing, check out the first chapter, Basics of Gym Climbing, which will give you general guidelines on how to use the gym, including etiquette, grades, resting, nutrition, safety, and warming up. If you'd rather explore exercises by what you want to train for or how much time you have, check out our Index of Exercises on page 242.

Games!

With hours spent pulling the same plastic holds and projecting the same problems, you might get a bit bored, so you'll find games sprinkled throughout the book. The lighthearted, competitive spirit and try-hard atmosphere of climbing in a group will get you psyched up, and you'll benefit from getting more time on the wall and taking a break from the "work" aspect of training. Get your friends and training partners involved and try these out a few times a week to stay inspired and enthusiastic—after all, the best climber in the world is the one having the most fun.

Note: Climbing outside is a completely different activity that requires a level of professional instruction this book will not provide. This book does not cover climbing outside. The good news is that your climbing gym is a great place to start. Ask at the front desk for classes on how to transition to outdoor climbing.

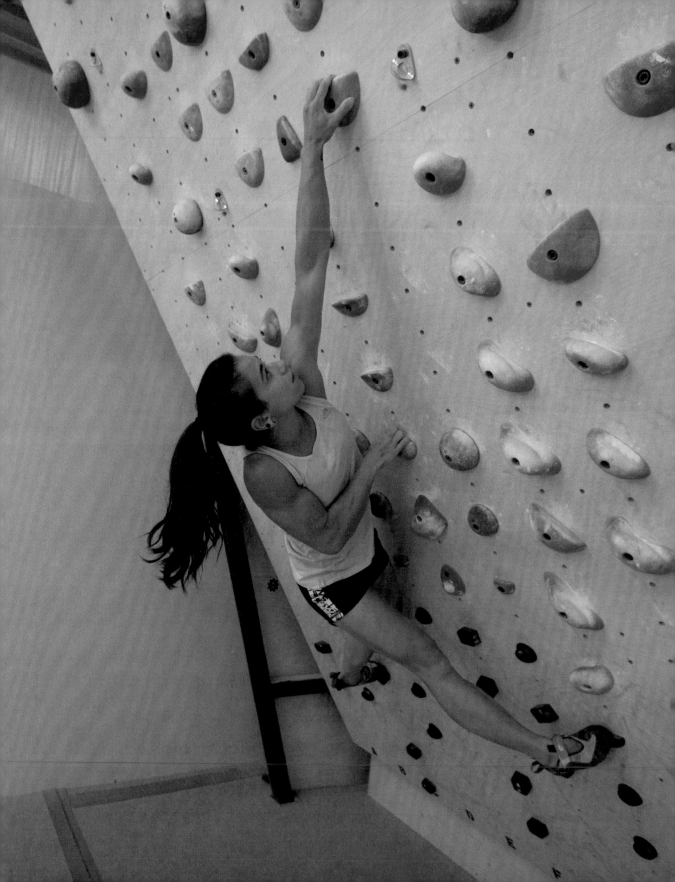

Chapter 1

BASICS OF GYM CLIMBING

YOU DON'T HAVE TO BE A PRO to have a great workout in a climbing gym. Don't worry if you're not very familiar with the ins and outs of gyms. This chapter offers all the information you need to maximize use of the climbing gym in your personal workout regimen. It includes information on roped climbing versus bouldering, grades, rest and recovery, nutrition basics, general guidelines for climbing in the gym, and etiquette. We'll also cover proper falling technique for bouldering and roped climbing, spotting for bouldering, and the correct warm-up.

ROPED CLIMBING VERSUS BOULDERING

This book contains an equal mix of roped climbing and bouldering workouts. Roped climbing, which includes toprope and lead, is just what it sounds like: You climb longer routes while tied into a rope, either with the rope running above you (a toprope) or from below (a lead). This is more of an endurance-based discipline, where you must stay on the wall longer. Generally the individual moves are easier, and the challenge comes when you do all those moves in a row without rest.

Conversely, bouldering is where you climb without a rope on much shorter walls. Typically this is a more power- and strength-focused discipline, where the individual moves are harder. Because you have to do fewer moves at one time, endurance is less of an issue, but pure strength is very important.

It doesn't matter which discipline you want to focus on—it all comes down to personal preference. In your own workouts, you might enjoy the challenge of figuring out longer routes and climbing with a partner, or you might like the solitary aspect

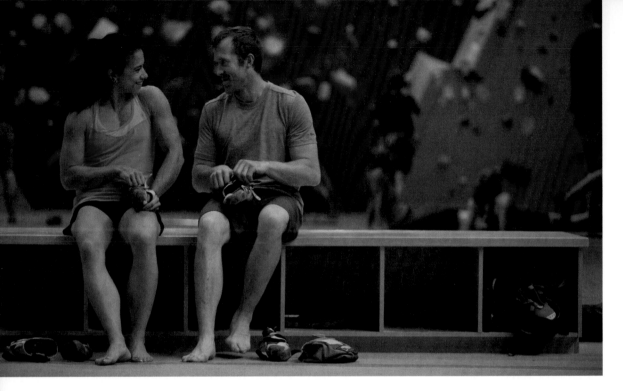

of bouldering and its more gymnastic, powerful movement. You might like both equally, or go through phases during which you want to focus on one or the other. That's great! Both types of climbing will make you stronger and more physically fit, and ultimately both disciplines require strength and endurance—they're not mutually exclusive.

NUTRITION

For any training or fitness program, it's absolutely crucial to keep your body fueled properly to promote muscle recovery, burn fat, and maintain energy. You can work out as much as you want, but if you don't eat the right food, your improvements will be limited. Research suggests that when you're trying to lose weight, burn fat, or build muscle, nutrition is at least 80 percent of success, while working out comprises 20 percent or less. Here are some healthy guidelines to follow:

▶ Maintain a healthy, balanced diet that's filled with natural foods, like lean meats, a *ton* of vegetables, whole grains, and fruit.

▶ Be wary of food that comes in any sort of package, box, or bag.

▶ Try to cut out excess sugar, fat, and processed foods.

- ▶ Opt for a good mix of protein, fat, and carbohydrates.

- ▶ Drink more water than you think you need: a minimum of 64 ounces per non-training day and 96 ounces on training days.

Because you will likely spend more than an hour at the climbing gym on any given day, it's important to fuel your body before, during, and after a workout. Eat carbohydrate like fruit about thirty minutes before training. Make sure it's something easy to digest that won't weigh you down or make you feel bloated. Do the same during your workout, eating a few bites of something every forty-five minutes or so. Within thirty to forty-five minutes after your workout, aim to get a mix of carbohydrates and protein to help rebuild muscles; a protein drink is a great solution. Your body is super receptive to these nutrients right after a workout, so try to get it within that timeframe. Once you've had your post-workout drink, try to eat a solid meal—again, with a good mix of carbs and protein—within about ninety minutes.

Understanding Macronutrients

Every calorie you consume can be broken down into a macronutrient category: carbohydrates, protein, or fat. They all play an important role in your health and performance. Below are general guidelines regarding how much of each maconutrient to consume, but be aware that your body might have specific requirements. Talk to a dietitian or nutritionist to figure out the unique needs of your body.

- ▶ **Carbohydrates (4 calories per gram, 55–65 percent of diet)**: Carbohydrates are fuel that we can't store a lot of. They're much more efficient at producing large amounts of energy in a limited time than fat. Carbs are important for aerobic and anaerobic training. If you burn carbohydrates aerobically, you will produce about twice as much energy per molecule as you would from fat.

- ▶ **Fats (9 calories per gram, 15–30 percent of diet)**: Fats are another fuel, and we're always burning fat, even when our bodies are at rest. Fat is the most efficient energy system, and you have an unlimited supply of it. You can get more out of each fat molecule than any other macronutrient—just not in a short amount of time. Fat has a small structural role in creating hormones, and it's part of our cell membranes; we need dietary fat just to keep our bodies healthy.

▶ **Protein (4 calories per gram, 15–25 percent of diet)**: Protein is not a fuel source, but athletes still benefit from eating a lot of it. It's primarily structural material, not just for your muscles but for your entire body. Basically, to some extent, everything in your body is made out of protein. We need to support our bodies with dietary protein. About 20 grams every three hours, through food or protein powder, is the ideal amount to maximize absorption.

GRADES

Climbs are given a number rating, called a grade, to denote difficulty. Some gyms use their own unique grading system, but typically boulder problems are graded on the V scale (see "grade" in the glossary, page 251) and roped climbs on the Yosemite Decimal System (YDS). The V scale starts with VB or V0 being the easiest;

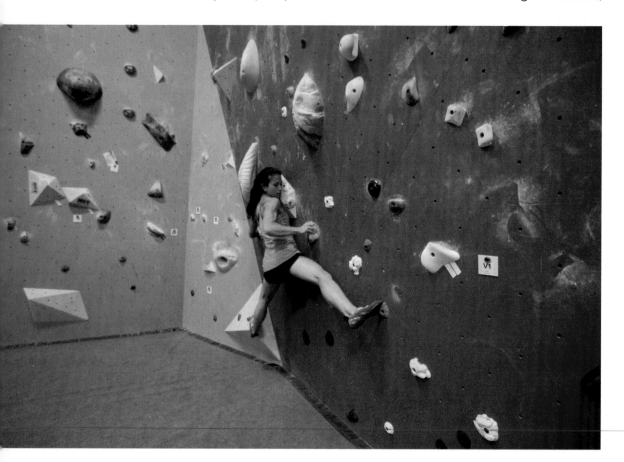

V1 is harder, V2 harder than V1, and so on. It's an open-ended scale, and the world's current hardest boulder problem is thought to be V17. The YDS starts at 5.0, and moves up as follows: 5.1, 5.2, 5.3, 5.4, etc. Once the grade reaches 5.7 and higher, a plus (+) or minus (−) can be added to further categorize difficulty. So, for example, 5.9− is easier than 5.9, which is easier than 5.9+. Some gyms use letter notations starting at 5.10 instead of the plus/minus system: 5.10a, 5.10b, 5.10c, and 5.10d are all 5.10, with 5.10a being the easiest and 5.10d being the hardest. Typically, a 5.10− is about the same as a 5.10a or 5.10b; 5.10 is 5.10b or 5.10c; and 5.10+ is 5.10c or 5.10d.

Grades are very subjective, and a 5.10 might feel easier than a 5.8. Some climbs might suit your height, body type, and strengths better than others. You might be able to grip small holds all day on a 5.11, but a 5.10 with big, rounded holds gives you difficulty. Typically, the routesetters who create the climbs suggest the grades, and then ask other climbers in the gym to offer input on the difficulty before settling on a final number. While grades are an excellent way to measure progress, or to choose a climb when training, don't get too caught up in chasing numbers.

GYM ETIQUETTE

All gyms have a formal set of rules, probably posted somewhere in the facility. Obviously you should follow those closely, but there is also a set of unspoken rules in the climbing gym, otherwise known as "climbing gym etiquette." Because there are only a certain number of routes or problems, there is a right and wrong way to approach how you queue up to climb. Below are some general etiquette suggestions.

▶ Avoid hogging routes if you can, but be aware that sometimes training requires you to climb the same route or problem multiple times. If that's the case, make sure whoever is waiting in line to go after you knows your plan. Communicate clearly and politely that you're training and will be on the route for a while. If you are the person waiting, thank the climber and move on, or wait quietly. If a group is taking its time, don't hesitate to ask them if they will be there for a while. The most common way to get in line for a roped route is to wait at the base.

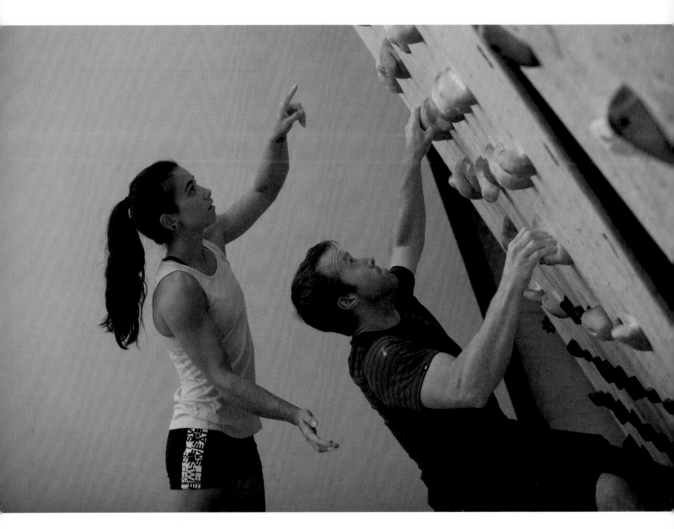

▶ Have good etiquette when waiting for a bouldering problem to open, and be mindful of those waiting around you. Because there's not usually a clear-cut line for each climb, communicate with the other climbers about getting on the wall. Above all else, don't be the rude person who jumps in front every time. Before you hop on the wall, make sure the holds you'll use don't interfere with another climb that someone might already be on. Some people like to brush holds to remove excess chalk, usually right before they climb. Don't get on a climb right after it's been brushed, unless the brusher explicitly offers it.

▶ If a boulderer seems to be struggling high off the ground, or is in a precarious position and looks like she might take a bad fall, don't be afraid to jump in and give her a respectful spot. Say out loud to the climber, "I've got your spot." It might give her the confidence she needs to fire the move and, if not, it will give her the assistance she needs for a safe landing.

▶ Don't offer unwarranted beta to other climbers, meaning don't give unsolicited information on how to complete a climb. It's common for climbers who are working on the same problems to talk about specific movements or holds, and help each other figure out how to get to the top, but ask if someone wants beta first. Many climbers enjoy the process of figuring out the problem on their own, so don't be the person who walks around talking about how you completed the climb.

REST AND RECOVERY

Rest is absolutely critical to getting stronger, both for overall and for climbing specifically. The key is finding the balance between pushing hard and exhausting your

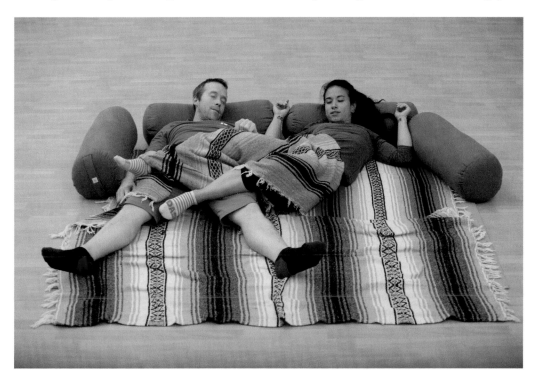

body, and resting enough so that your muscles and systems can recover. That downtime is when your body rebuilds itself. Listen to your body; if anything feels tweaked or painful, don't focus your workout on that area.

Pay attention to the difference between a full rest day and an active rest day. If you are training moderately, consider taking active rest days—when you ride your bike, jog, or hike at a leisurely pace. These active rest days are excellent for cross-training, in which you work different body systems than climbing works, so focus on light cardio, stretching, yoga, and other antagonist exercises. If you're training seriously and feel totally wrecked, take a full rest day and don't do anything.

With training and resting, consistency is key. Pick a weekly schedule that works for you and is easy to stick to. For the sake of this book, weekly schedules start on Mondays, but you can adjust these schedules to best fit your needs. Aim to climb three days in a week, or even four if you want, but don't climb more than two days in a row. If you push really hard one climbing day, consider taking the next day off. Climb Monday, Wednesday, and Friday, with Tuesday and Thursday as rest days. Or climb two days on, one day off, two days on, one day off, two days on, four days off, then repeat. Resting is one of the most important things you can do, as it allows your muscles time to recover and strengthen, and for you to come back refreshed and reenergized. Take your rest days and recovery time just as seriously as you do climbing or training time.

Another body part that is important to rest is your skin. The texture on climbing holds can turn the skin on your palms and fingers red and raw, especially when you first start climbing. The more often you climb, the more that skin will harden and turn into calluses. This thicker skin will withstand the abuses of climbing better, but make sure to take at least a few days off every week so your skin can rest and regrow.

GENERAL GUIDELINES

Climbing in the gym might seem like a pretty straightforward activity, but there are some important guidelines everyone should follow to stay healthy and safe. This is just a starting point, so make sure to check if your gym has its own rules.

▶ **Always warm up thoroughly before climbing**. You don't want to go from zero to sixty and end up with an injury, so climb easy terrain for about fifteen minutes, then incorporate progressively smaller holds on a few moves here and there.

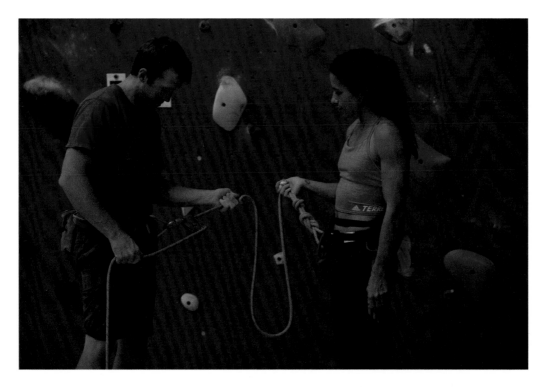

Get your body ready to climb by doing a few easy routes, jumping jacks, jogging, stretching, etc. Cool down after workouts by climbing a final few easy routes/ problems, and by stretching. This will help you avoid injury and promote recovery. You can also do a series of dynamic stretches, or check out our suggestion for the Perfect Warm-Up on page 23.

▶ **Don't walk directly under other climbers or get in the way of their belayers**. The same goes for when you're on the wall: keep an eye on whomever or what- ever is underneath you, and don't try any difficult moves, where you might fall off, if there's anyone near your landing. Don't distract belayers when they're belaying. That means waiting until a climber is done before asking a question or chatting. It is each climber's personal responsibility to keep himself or herself safe, but you should also be looking out for others' safety. Don't be afraid to comment politely if someone is doing something that looks dangerous, or ask a gym staffer to intervene.

▶ **When roped climbing, always perform safety checks with your partner**. Make sure her harness is positioned properly and tightened securely, with the buckles doubled back. She should do the same with you. Confirm that her tie-in knot is threaded through both tie-in points, tied, and dressed correctly. Your partner should confirm that your belay device is set up according to manufacturer instructions and that the carabiner is locked. Note: If you do not know what this means, seek professional instruction. When using an autobelay, double- and triple-check that you are clipped in properly. Most accidents with autobelays occur when the climber completely forgets to clip in, which can occur when you're distracted or don't have a partner to check you.

▶ **Communication between partners when roped climbing is paramount.** As the belayer, you should pay attention to the climber, taking in and feeding out slack appropriately. Don't be afraid to call up to the climber, and vice versa to the belayer. If either cannot understand the other due to loud music or general noise, consider moving to another area of the gym. That also means not wearing headphones when climbing or belaying!

▶ **Remove all jewelry (rings, bracelets, long necklaces, and earrings) and take everything out of your pockets.** There should be nothing hanging off your body that could injure you or your spotter when you fall.

▶ **Don't climb higher than you're comfortable with**, whether that's 5 feet or 15 feet, and keep in mind your gym's specific rules. Some gyms have standalone boulders to top out on, meaning you climb up and over, finishing on top of the wall. Other boulders might not be made for topping out; instead you'll touch the top and drop off or downclimb. Some boulder problems are at the base of taller, roped climbing walls, where there's a sign or tape marking the maximum height allowed for bouldering.

▶ **Don't leave anything out on the mats where falling climbers might land.** That includes chalk bags, water bottles, shoes, keys, phones, etc.

▶ **Follow the rules of your specific gym**. These might include no loose chalk, no gear on the pads, no street shoes on the mat, no climbing above a certain height, etc.

THE PERFECT WARM-UP

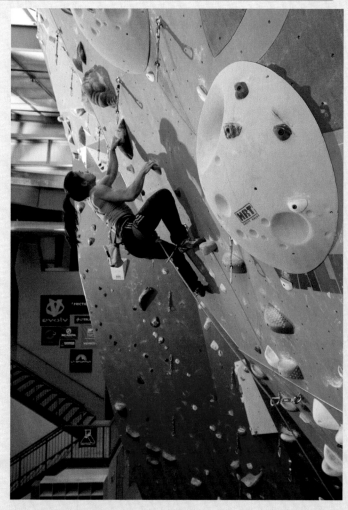

You might be tempted to skip the proper pre-climb procedures. However, getting your body ready to work hard is an essential step, plus it will make your whole climbing session more efficient and effective. "Ready to send" is an essential step. Not enough warm-up, and you might end up with a killer flash-pump (swollen forearms from hell) on that onsight burn or, worse, a brutal finger injury. Overdo it, and you might be too fatigued to effectively train or climb. If you don't already have your own tried-and-true warm-up ritual, consider incorporating the following suggestions into your routine to prepare your body for success. These pointers will ease you into send-mode with confidence.

1 GET THE BLOOD MOVING. Ten minutes of walking, biking, or jogging get the heart circulating blood around the body while simultaneously warming up the often-overlooked leg muscles. Try to spend at least five minutes on your feet, walking around to check out different climbs or saying hi to friends. Some light cardio improves circulation and starts delivering blood and oxygen to all the muscles in your body, stoking them with the fuel necessary to perform. Try the treadmill, or consider walking or biking to the gym.

2 LOOSEN UP. The classic concept of stretching involves holding a certain pose for fifteen to thirty seconds, but sports science research shows that this form of static stretching actually decreases muscle output. Instead, dynamic stretching with rotational movements offers more benefit to muscles by adding an element of momentum to flexibility, and by simulating the types of strain muscles undergo while climbing. Biologically, dynamic stretches lube up the joints and tendons vital to climbing, which increases muscle performance and reduces the risk of injury. Static stretching is useful on rest days or after activity as a supplementary tool to improve overall flexibility. We recommend a few minutes of the following stretches to kick up your session.

▶ **Head Rolls:** These are especially good for steep climbing, where you'll be craning your neck to look up, and for boulderers who will be falling and jarring their necks and upper backs from impact with the mats. Let your head completely relax forward, then slowly roll your head in a circle, five times in both directions. Keep it as loose as possible all the way around to really stretch and awaken those muscles. This will also help align the vertebrae in your back to prevent injuries.

▶ **Windmills:** Keeping your arms straight, swing them slowly in a circle, making sure to rotate at the shoulders. Keep the circles controlled the whole way around. Go five times in both directions, one arm at a time. Next, put your arms straight out and do smaller, more controlled circles (just a few inches around), forward then backward. Do both arms at once. Shoulders are among the most commonly injured joints among climbers, and can be ignored on easy routes.

These stretches focus on your shoulder joints while sending blood to muscles in your forearms and fingers.

▶ **Side Twists:** Lie down with your feet on the floor and knees bent. Lift your upper body slightly off the ground with your hands on your stomach. Rotate your upper body slowly and deliberately from side to side, engaging your abdominals. This shouldn't feel like a full-on ab workout, but will instead lightly engage your core right off the bat. Aim for twisting to each side at least five times, rest a minute, and repeat.

▶ **Walking Lunges:** These will get your lower body and core ready to climb. Keeping your body upright, step forward with one leg and slowly drop until your lunging leg's knee is a few inches off the ground. As you stand back up, smoothly step forward with the other leg, and drop into the next lunge. Repeat until you've done about ten lunges on each leg.

3 **PYRAMID CLIMBING.** Now that your blood is pumping, your joints are limber, and your body is ready to work, it's time to climb. While most people understand they need to start with climbs well under their limit, the best warm-up sequence actually builds in difficulty up to just under your personal maximum. The first problem or route should fall well within your ability. For instance, a V5 boulderer should start with several V1s and V2s. The goal of the first problem is both to engage all the little muscle groups used in climbing and to mentally refresh good technique. If the first climb feels at all strenuous, immediately drop down a grade. After resting about five minutes, get on a few problems that are slightly harder than the first round: two to three grades under your limit for boulderers. For example, the V5 boulderer should work a V3. Rest another few minutes—enough to fully depump—and get on your final warm-up climb of the day: something right below your limit. (See also V4 Boulderer Pyramid Warm-Up, page 27.)

4 **REST.** After this warm-up sequence, it's important to rest properly, but be careful not to cool down too much, which will lead you to the dreaded flash-pump, in which your forearms swell with blood and lactic acid, leaving you too weak to hold onto the wall even when you should be feeling fresh. A ten-minute final rest should suffice.

PROPER BOULDERING FALLS

One of the true joys of bouldering lies in its simplicity, which also makes it an excellent introduction to the sport of climbing. There are no complicated rope systems, you typically don't get too high off the ground, and all you really need is climbing shoes and some chalk.

Bouldering seems safer than other forms of climbing, but the short falls are high impact and can easily lead to injury if you hit the pads wrong. Feeling comfortable falling on pads will also help you focus on trying hard on the wall, instead of being

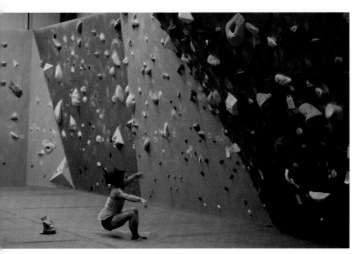

scared of hitting the ground. Knowing how to fall safely and land softly helps prevent injury, so incorporate a few practice falls into your warm-up routine, or throughout your gym session. There's a saying in climbing: "If you're not falling, you're not trying hard enough." As you get more comfortable with falling, you'll have more confidence to push past your limits. Eventually, a safe falling technique will become engrained as muscle memory.

Following Guidelines

No two falls are exactly the same, and the gymnastic moves of bouldering often put our bodies in awkward positions, meaning there's no "one true way" when it comes to safer landings. The following are guidelines to practice any time you head out for a bouldering session.

▶ Before you pull onto the wall, scope the landing zone to make sure it's free of everything, from water bottles and chalk bags to other climbers.

▶ Once you start to peel off, never try to grab other holds to catch yourself. Accept that you're falling and go with the flow—literally. The key is to find a good balance between keeping your whole body slightly engaged and yet also somewhat relaxed. This might sound impossible, but finding the sweet spot of keeping muscles activated but soft is the key to safe landings. Tensing up too much before impact will lead to strains, sprains, and even bone breaks, not to mention ligament injuries and muscle tears.

▶ Try to land with a shoulder-width or wider stance and bent, soft knees, directing most of the impact into your strong lower body, which is designed to absorb that sort of falling force.

▶ Land with the bottoms of your feet squarely on the mat, instead of the heels, toes, or sides of the feet.

▶ Tucking your chin to your chest will help engage your neck muscles to prevent whiplash, which is a common injury for boulderers, especially after falling from a horizontal roof.

▶ When you land, allow your self to tuck in and roll down onto your side, back, or shoulder. Don't fight the momentum of the fall; allow it to take you down to the mat in a soft "tuck and roll" manner.

▶ Never try to stop yourself with your hands or arms. Landing on an outstretched hand or arm can lead to upper-extremity injuries like sprains, strains, or breaks. As you're falling, try to hug your arms high and into your chest. This prevents you from instinctively reaching your arms down to stop a fall, and it keeps them out of the way so you won't bash them on any obstacles on your way down.

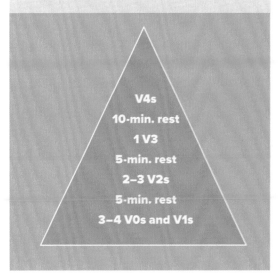

V4 BOULDERER PYRAMID WARM-UP

If you're going to be bouldering for the day, consider this bouldering pyramid warm-up, where you start at the bottom. The idea is to start off easy and do more climbing at that level, rest a bit, then move on to slightly harder climbs, rest, and so on.

V4s
10-min. rest
1 V3
5-min. rest
2–3 V2s
5-min. rest
3–4 V0s and V1s

▶ When falling from a low roof where your body is almost horizontal, keep your arms and legs elevated, almost like they're still holding onto the wall, allowing your back to absorb the impact (think of a turtle flipped over onto its shell). Remember to tuck your chin to your chest to prevent whiplash.

▶ Dynos can cause scary, face-down falls that leave little time to correct your body position. Keep arms and legs up to avoid landing on them, and turn your head to one side to stabilize the neck and prevent whiplash. Try to engage your core as well, to soften the landing.

▶ When landing directly on your back or stomach, instead of curling your arms up into your chest, try to slap the mat out to your sides at the moment of impact. This will counteract the force of the fall and engage your upper body just enough to keep it from flopping around, which can cause injury.

Bouldering Spotting Technique

Gyms with fully padded floors in the bouldering area rarely require a spotter, but some gyms still use movable crash pads, and even fully padded gyms might have

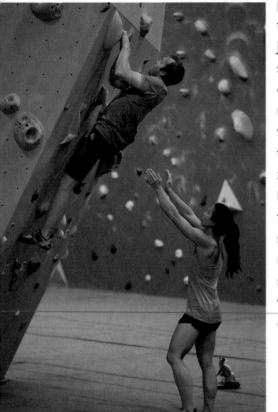

problems that climb over an unpadded zone. In those instances you'll need a spotter. The spotter's job is to guide the climber's body so it lands in the safest spot possible. That doesn't mean catching the climber; instead, the spotter should have her arms up, elbows bent, and wrists and hands soft, ready to grasp the falling climber's hips or waist and gently push her toward the safest part of the landing zone while simultaneously protecting her climber's head and neck. A good spot relies on a good stance: feet a little more than shoulder-width apart, one foot slightly in front of the other with knees bent. Take the role of spotting seriously, and, when climbing, pick a spotter you trust, so you don't have to worry about who's got your back. You will be able to try your hardest without thinking about the ground below you.

5 BASIC RULES FOR SPOTTING

1 **COMMUNICATION.** Before anyone leaves the ground, both the climber and spotter need clarity. As a climber, never assume you're spotted. Check before you start up. As a spotter, it's critical to talk with your climber about likely falls, and what to do in case of a planned dismount versus an unexpected fall. Know which problem your climber intends to try, including any cruxes, bad holds, or dynamic moves.

2 **PAD ARRANGEMENT.** Many climbing gyms have fully padded floors with no gaps between pads, but some gyms use movable crash pads. In the latter scenario, boulderers can roll ankles on poorly placed pads, so watch for gaps, tangle-prone straps, sharp objects, and uneven landing zones. You'll sometimes need to move pads on the fly to match your climber's fall, but plan first by identifying potential fall spots to avoid any disastrous last-minute shuffles. Never take a pad out from under a climber while she's on the wall.

3 **SPOTTER'S STANCE.** Start with the correct stance: Stand closely behind your climber with your elbows crooked and hands by his waist. Put your dominant foot forward and slightly bend your knees. Discern where the climber might fall, especially with an uneven landing zone or big, dynamic movements. And be ready to move quickly. Also, focus on your climber and not your smartphone or the sandwich waiting in your pack. A good rule of thumb is to train your eyes on a point high on the back of your climber's shirt.

4 **SIZE DIFFERENCE.** When spotting, being taller than and/or outweighing your climber is not mandatory. In most cases, your goal is simply to steer the falling climber onto a pad. Do this from your active stance by pushing the climber's center of gravity—usually hips for gals, waist for boys—toward the pad while also protecting the neck and head.

5 **THUMBS IN OR OUT.** Some prefer thumbs out, separate from the palm, while others suggest thumbs pressed against the hand. Critics of the thumbs-out method say that you can easily break your thumb if it catches on the falling climber. Critics of the thumbs-in method say that it's much easier to guide the force of a falling climber with the thumbs-out method. Find what works for you, and stick with it.

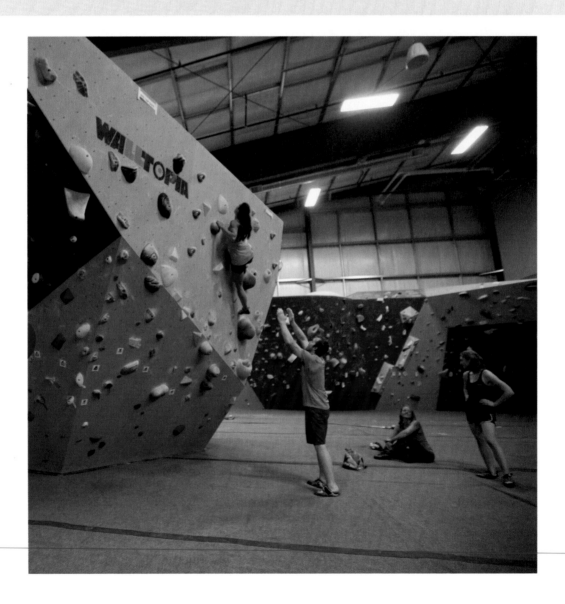

FALLING ON A ROPE

Falling is essential for advancing as a climber—it's a key part of the sport, at any fitness level. To progress, you must try moves that are at the edge of your ability—or beyond—and when you try that hard, you will fall. Every climber falls, even the world's best. Toprope falls are the safest, but falling also can be quite safe on well-protected lead climbs, as long as you have good technique and a solid belayer. Before climbing into a situation where you may take a leader fall, assess the dangers, including corners, arêtes, protruding holds, or other climbers below that you might hit.

Falling Practice

Falling is a skill, and practice makes you better. "Practice falls" can ease the jitters before a hard climb, or cure a long-term case of the heebie-jeebies.

▶ Choose a sport climb up a vertical or gently overhanging face.

▶ Enlist an experienced belayer. You want someone you can be confident in, and who has experience.

▶ Choose a spot at least 35 to 40 feet up so there's more stretch in the rope system to absorb the impact and there's no chance of a ground fall.

▶ Start out with a few falls on toprope (meaning you're climbing on lead, but you've clipped a bolt above your head). Then fall with your tie-in knot six inches above the bolt, then a foot, then two feet. Focus on the "Dos" of good falling technique.

▶ Practice frequently to imprint muscle (and mental!) memory.

How to Fall (Bouldering and Roped)

DO

▶ Warn your belayer if you think you might fall. Yell, "Watch me here!"

▶ Shout "Falling!" as you peel off.

▶ Look straight down to spot your landing and any obstacles. This also leads to the best body position for a safe fall.

▶ Breathe out to help relax the body. Shrieking counts, though you may lose a few style points.

▶ Relax your legs. Keep your arms and legs slightly bent, with your knees "soft" and ready to absorb any impact. Think falling like a cat.

▶ Keep your hands up, forward, and a little out to the sides, for better balance and to avoid scraping them on the wall or catching them in the rope. Let your legs absorb the impact when you swing into the wall.

DON'T

▶ Fall with the rope behind your foot or leg. That can give you nasty rope burn or even flip you upside down, cracking your head against the wall. As you're climbing, stay aware of how the rope is running; your belayer should help by alerting you if you're climbing with the rope behind your leg. Keep it in front of your legs and feet (rope running off the tie-in points and over one hip), or between them, especially near the start of a route, when pulling past an overhang, and when clipping. If you're traversing, avoid stepping such that your body is between the rope and the wall—thread your foot behind the rope instead, so it stays in front of you. If the rope ends up behind your legs or ankles, take the time to step around it and reposition.

▶ Push off the wall as you fall, unless you're an experienced climber who can see that shoving off might help you clear a ledge or another obstacle below. Pushing off just throws your body out of balance and puts you in position to slam back into the wall when the rope comes tight.

▶ Grab anything to try and stop yourself. Grabbing a quickdraw, bolt, or the rope is a recipe for rope burn or a severely injured finger. (Many climbers have lost digits this way.) Let the rope and belayer do their jobs without interference.

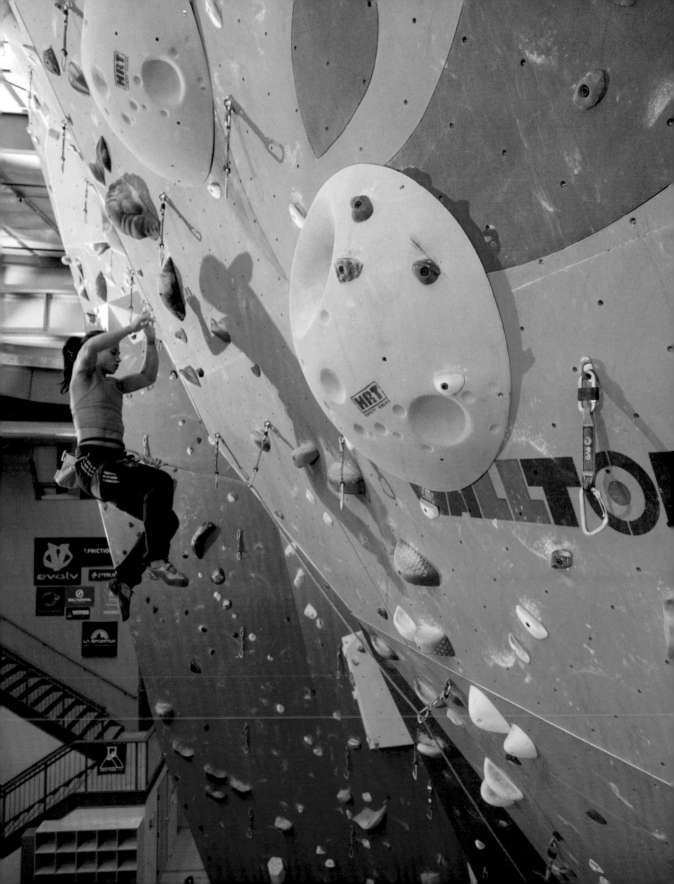

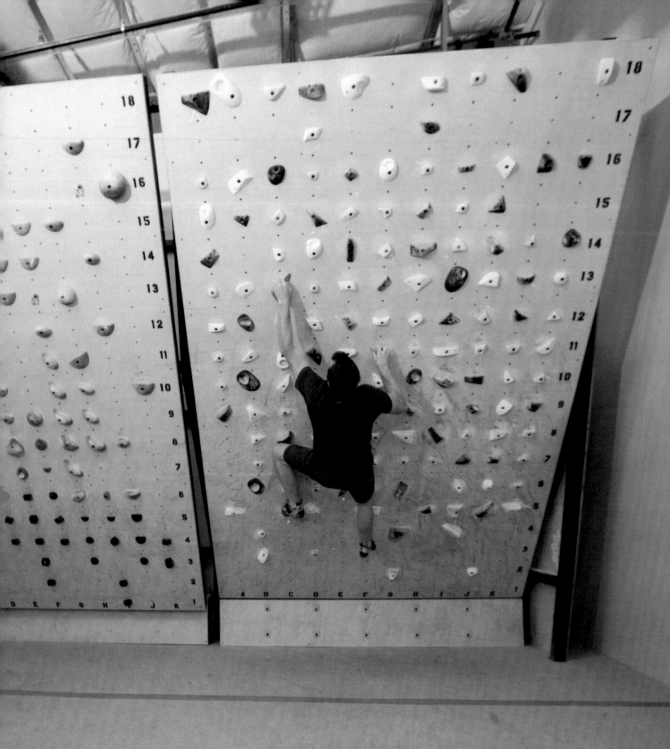

Chapter 2

STRENGTH

STRENGTH IS THE ABILITY TO PERFORM A SPECIFIC MOVE with your body, whether it's a long reach or gripping small holds. You must have strength in your legs to push, in your arms to pull, in your forearms and fingers to hold on, and in your core to pull it all together. When you first start climbing, you'll see your overall strength increase rapidly, as muscles you've never used before are suddenly asked to do difficult tasks. (Hello, burning forearms!)

All types of climbing will increase your strength, but bouldering targets strength in a more direct way than roped climbing, which also focuses on endurance. You'll perform many of the following workouts on the bouldering wall to hone in on increasing strength. If you're familiar with weight training, think of strength building in bouldering as a "low rep, high weight" style, where you focus on moving heavy weights a handful of times. Strength building with roped climbing would be more akin to "high rep, low weight."

Another main aspect to bouldering is power, or the speed at which you can generate strength for certain moves. Bouldering walls are shorter, usually 12 to 20 feet high, and the individual moves are usually more difficult. Movement sequences can be cryptic, which provides a fun problem-solving element. Each climber must figure out how to do moves and link sequences that suit his or her unique strength and size.

While you won't need a climbing partner for bouldering, this type of climbing can be quite social, as most of your time will be spent standing on the ground with other people who are trying the same climbs. Some climbers enjoy this aspect, as it makes going to the gym quite fun, while others might prefer more focused training. It will come down to personal preference—whether you like to try hard in short spurts (bouldering), or if you prefer to stay on the wall for longer times (roped climbing). However, it's important to remember that training strength will help with both types of climbing, versus training endurance, which is more geared toward climbing on ropes. If you're looking to get strong, build power, or develop a muscular physique, read on.

BOULDERING INTERVALS

The focus of this exercise is power-endurance, or the halfway point between power (the ability to generate strength quickly) and endurance (the ability to maintain that power for longer periods). In bouldering, this translates to being able to do many hard moves in a row, without getting pumped to the point where you fall off. Similar to other training intervals, the goal is to work really hard for short periods of time, and then to rest completely and recover as much as possible. This is a great fat-burning workout.

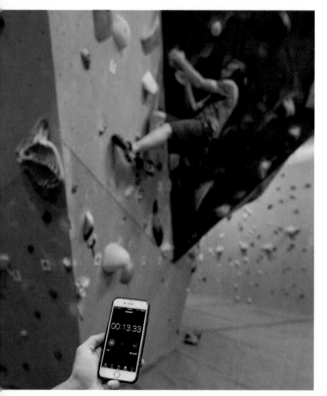

▶ *Bouldering Intervals*

The Workout

You'll need a stopwatch and a partner. The goal is to ascend five strenuous boulder problems in five minutes with minimal resting. The climbs should be challenging and near your limit, so it's OK to fall here and there. They should be easy to descend, meaning you can drop off quickly and safely once you reach the top. This minimizes recovery time, which is important for honing in on power-endurance. Remember, you only have five minutes to do five problems. Once the five minutes are up (regardless of whether you've sent all five problems), it's your turn to be timer/spotter while your partner goes. Do three (beginner) to six (advanced) rounds of these bouldering intervals. Make a game of it by keeping score and determining a winner of each round by adding up the V numbers of the five problems completed.

PROJECT, PUSH-UP, PULL-UP

Power, an essential part of bouldering, can be difficult to attain by just climbing on the wall, but a simple way is to try big moves on good holds when you're already tired. This forces your mind and your muscles to dig deep and find that extra *oomph* to get certain moves done, which will come in handy on every climb. It can also help you feel the difference between when you're trying and when you're trying *hard*. Even on easy problems, bouldering is all about the latter, and you might find you can do a lot more than you think if you just give it some "grr."

The Workout

Find a project at your limit that you've never been on, isn't your style (e.g., if you're bad at slopers, make sure it has slopers), and is something you wouldn't mind putting some effort into. Work on your project for fifteen minutes. When the time is up, you have five minutes to do 50 push-ups and 20 pull-ups.

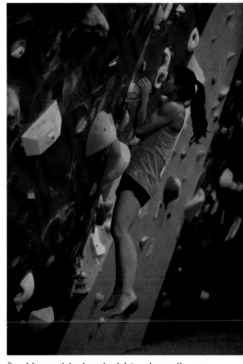

Even if you haven't done that many, quit when the five minutes is up. That's one round. Do six rounds of this: By the end, you will have put ninety minutes into your project and aimed for 300 push-ups and 120 pull-ups. It might take you a while to work up to doing that many, but keep pushing yourself! That's when you will see max improvement. Bring a notepad to keep track of your rounds.

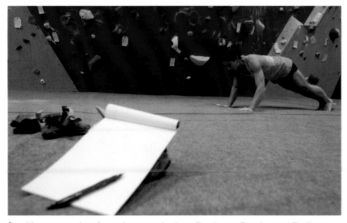

▶ *Keep track of push-ups during Project, Push-up, Pull-up.*

▶ *Use a big jug hold to do pull-ups for Project, Push-up, Pull-up.*

BOOKENDS

If you like to spend most of your training time on the wall, you'll find this exercise can improve your climbing immediately. This workout focuses on technique, or how precisely and efficiently you move on the wall, so consider doing this workout on a day when your body is feeling tired. Learning to optimally place your feet and then transfer your body weight onto them reduces the load on your forearms and puts your body in a position to reach the next set of handholds efficiently. Plus, the muscles in your legs are larger and have more stamina than those in your arms, so the more propulsion you get out of those quads, glutes, hamstrings, and calves, the better. The net result is climbing that feels anywhere from a little to a whole lot easier.

Below are some suggestions for dialing in technique—and if you do this at the same time you build strength, you'll become a drastically better climber. Pay attention to how your body feels (sensory feedback) while performing the drills, and practice them frequently. Your new skills won't become part of your on-the-wall repertoire unless they are natural and familiar. You can accelerate this by attempting these drills on increasingly difficult terrain.

The Workout

Start and end any climbing session with solid technique practice. This way, if you start to use improper or poor movement as you grow more fatigued, you're still reinforcing good technique at the end of the routine. After warming up, but before the climbing session, do ten to twenty minutes of specific technique drills (read on for suggestions) at a low intensity, with slow, methodical movements that emphasize flexibility. Do the same after climbing but before cooling down—hence the "bookends." The drills consist of doing the exact same movements five or more times in a row. You don't have to climb entire problems, just pull on the wall and find holds that force certain movements.

Below are drills you can incorporate into your workout.

PRECISION FEET

Goal: Toe accuracy

As you traverse on the bouldering wall, pick the optimal placement on every foothold you encounter, and move your foot onto this exact location with great precision, like a bull's-eye. Do not take your eyes off the foothold until your foot is perfectly placed. Move quicker as your skill level increases.

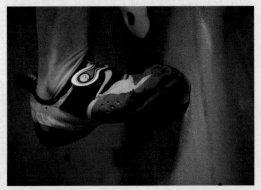 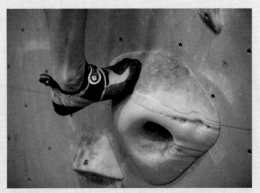

▶ *Practice Precision Feet on a variety of hold types.*

FOOT STAB

Goal: Improve coordination

With your climbing shoes on, stand in front of the wall and balance on one leg. Reach out and accurately touch preselected foothold targets with your raised foot. For increased difficulty, pick targets that require tricky reaches and challenge your balance.

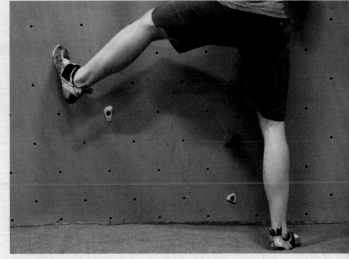

▶ *Foot Stab*

BLINKING

Goal: Evaluate foot placement by feel

Pick out a foothold and move your foot toward its exact location. Before your foot makes contact, close your eyes and finish locating the hold using spatial awareness. Keep your eyes closed until you have your foot securely placed. Evaluate your performance first through feel, and then open your eyes to confirm. Pick out the next hold and continue.

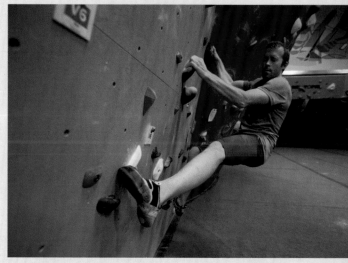
▶ *Blinking*

JIBS ONLY

Goal: Utilize bad holds

Only allow yourself to use the smallest footholds on the wall: tiny screw-on jibs, small divots in the wall, waves molded into the body of handholds, and natural features on the surface of the wall. This will teach you to use poor features accurately, which is often the case with technical climbs.

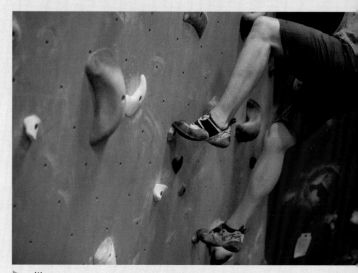
▶ *Jibs*

DOWNCLIMBING

Goal: Focus on lower extremities

Many people develop tunnel vision and focus only on what is directly above them and in reach. When they get stuck in this pattern, they tend to forget the hips, legs, and feet. Practice downclimbing, and let your feet lead the way as you shift your body to weight and utilize your feet most effectively.

GLUE FEET

Goal: Increase holding power and prevent slips

Imagine that your toes become frozen to the hold as soon as you place a foot; you can't change the relationship between foot and hold—no pivoting, tilting, or repositioning. All you're allowed to do is flex at the

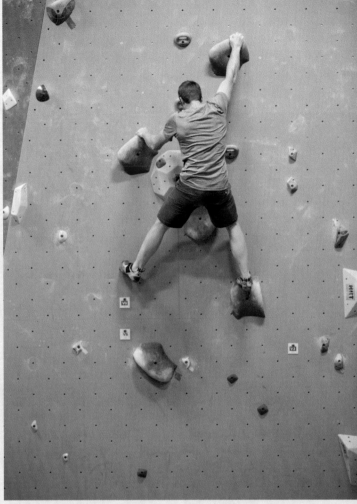

▶ *Downclimbing*

ankle when moving past the hold. Learn to establish and feel a wide contact area between your foot and the hold, and then work to maintain this maximum contact while the rest of your body moves.

OBSERVE

Goal: Learn from others

Watch advanced climbers on the exact route or boulder problem you just climbed. When in witness mode, analyze how they move and use their feet. Also, note which footholds they use and consider why. Another option is to watch World Cup competition climbing videos to glean footwork nuances that you can later practice yourself.

Drill Tips

▶ Wear tight-fitting, high-performance climbing shoes. Because these are the shoes you'll wear when you're trying your hardest climbs, wearing them for the footwork practice will help you understand what you can effectively stand on and move off of. Your "mileage" gym shoes will typically be too sloppy and loose to get the desired result and practice.

▶ Stay low to the ground so you can focus on the movement and not worry about falling.

▶ Keep your feet low and move them frequently. Most gym routes encourage large movements between footholds. While high-stepping or a wide stem may help you send the blue route, these techniques have much less value for trying to get better. When practicing, make small, frequent foot placements. Specifically, try making three foot placements for every hand move. Don't be surprised if you have to add intermediate feet that aren't part of the designated route. Climbing in this style trains you to keep your body centered and close to the wall, with your weight on your feet.

▶ Focus on feet and body, not hands. It's easy to get fixated on hand sequences and simply put your feet on the biggest holds you can find. The gym offers an excellent place to experiment with how utilizing different foothold locations can drastically affect body position, which in turn affects the use of handholds.

▶ Weight footholds correctly. There is more to good footwork than just putting your piggies exactly where you want them. Once your feet are in position, concentrate on wrapping your toes over the hold while weighting your foot in a way that maximizes friction between hold and rubber. This requires a large amount of core strength and body awareness.

LOCKOFFS

A lockoff is a static move in which you pull down hard on a hold with one hand until that arm is bent, then you hold that engaged position and reach up to another hold with your other arm. You're essentially "locking off" the first hold so you can complete the next move. This is essential in bouldering, where the holds are often widely spaced. Intermediate climbers can lock off near their shoulders and slightly below, while elite-level climbers can sometimes lock off at their waists. The stronger your lockoff strength (holding your arm in that position), the farther you can reach and the easier long, static moves will feel. If you're a shorter climber, lockoff strength becomes integral to progressing through the grades.

The Workout

Find a boulder or sport climb that you can do consistently—usually a few grades below your redpoint level. Climb the selected route and lock off every single move, holding the reaching hand just below the next hold for three seconds—count slowly or have someone else count while you climb. This will force you to focus on the intricacies, so that your body position has to be nearly perfect to efficiently execute. By the end of the climb, if you don't feel like you had to try hard, downclimb in the same fashion, pausing with the hand that's reaching down to the next hold. Rest a few minutes and move on to the next problem—do this for each climb, increasing the grade if you can.

PETER PANS

There are three things that will make you a better climber: core, core, and more core. Peter Pans are a great way to focus on core by just climbing—no need to get on the floor and crank out a thousand crunches or ten minutes of planks. Next time you get on the wall, imagine a line from your fingertips to your toes. You must keep every muscle in this line tight to stay on the wall. This is called body tension, and a strong core is crucial for maintaining it. The basic idea behind Peter Pans is to execute standard climbing moves, but intentionally remove your feet and swing them out from the wall (also called cutting your feet). Bouldering requires plenty of big, dynamic moves, where your feet will cut naturally, so this drill teaches you to react quickly and activate the correct muscles when this happens. Doing this on a rope builds incredible core endurance. This is also a great way to get worked if you don't have much time at the gym.

The Workout

Choose an overhanging climb with decent holds all the way up. Grade doesn't matter, as long as the holds are big and easy to grip; you shouldn't attempt this on tiny crimps or bad slopers. For each move, cut both feet intentionally. Swing your feet off the wall and then back on. Make the next move, and then swing them off the wall and back on. Repeat for every move on the climb. Keep your arms slightly bent to help engage your core; don't straight-arm anything. This workout will tire your entire body pretty quickly, so you might not need as many climbs to get worked. Beginners should aim for 10 problems when bouldering or 5 routes when roped climbing; intermediate/advanced climbers should aim for 15 to 20 problems, on 10 routes.

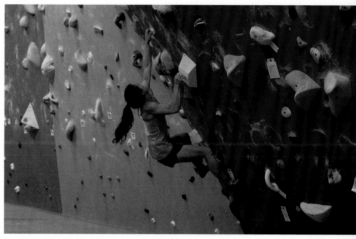

▶ *For Peter Pans, pick a slightly steep section of the wall.*

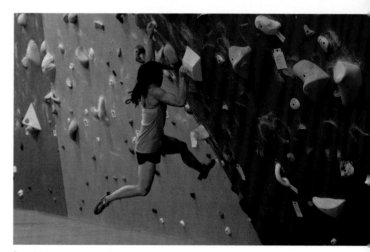

▶ *Between each move, purposely cut your feet and swing them back to the wall.*

WORLD CUP SIMULATOR

The World Cup series is a climbing competition in which the best climbers from each country compete on a series of bouldering problems. Because the competitors are top-tier athletes, the problems are extremely hard, and can have complicated or intricate sequences. There is also a time limit for each problem, which

Foothold Handbook

Here's how to get the best purchase on common gym holds:

Pocket

▶ Place pointed toe precisely in the opening

▶ Press down with forefoot

▶ Raise heel slightly to engage calf

Flat Wall

▶ Smear like on a slab

▶ Drop heel as far as possible to maximize contact

▶ Bend toes upward to engage forefoot

Small Edge

▶ Focus on the most positive part of the edge

▶ Keep ankle at about 90 degrees

▶ Wrap toes around hold; drive outside edge of big toe down onto hold

Sloper

▶ Drop heel to maximize contact

▶ Push toes and forefoot down

▶ Stay up high on hold

restricts the amount of rest a climber can get and creates an extra element of pressure. This exercise mimics that format, so you will have to keep your mental focus sharp as your body tires. You must execute under pressure while building power and endurance.

The Workout

Pick a project you know you'd have to work on for at least one full gym session before sending it. Project that boulder problem for 15 minutes by trying it from the

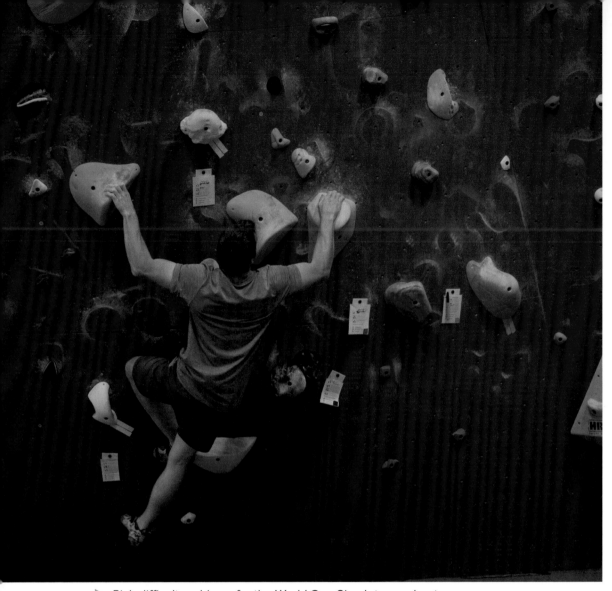

▶ *Pick difficult problems for the World Cup Simulator workout.*

bottom until you reach a move that stumps you, then continue working from that move upward until you figure it out. Once this 15-minute round is up, you have 15 minutes to climb every problem in the gym of a certain grade. That's one set. For example, say you pick a V4 that you know will be difficult. Work that for 15 minutes. Then climb every V1 in the gym within 15 minutes (at least five problems). If you fail at completing every problem, move on to the next project round. Do six sets of this. Rests will be in between attempts on the project. If you send the project before six rounds, pick another project and complete the sets with the new problem.

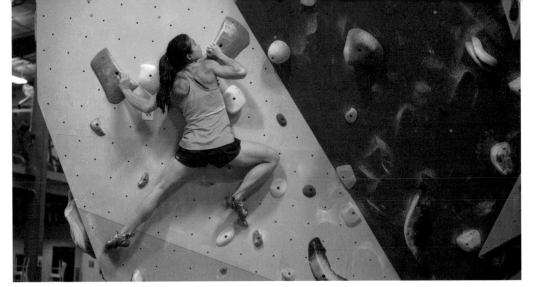
▶ *Flash Sessions*

ONSIGHT SESSIONS

The goal of this exercise is to onsight a series of problems, meaning climb all of them the first time without falling and with no prior knowledge of the moves. This is a great workout to do when the bouldering wall has just been reset. This will develop your onsighting ability, meaning the skill it takes to read climbs from the ground and while on the wall, to know how to grab particular holds, and to know how to move off them. The better you get at it, the more your overall climbing will improve. During the workout, resting time will be limited, so it's also a great way to build endurance quickly, as well as power-endurance. You'll repeat the same problems multiple times; this helps develop muscle memory, and your body will go through the motions with minimal involvement from your mind. The more you climb, the more individual moves become engrained in your muscle memory.

The Workout

Identify five challenging problems that you can feasibly onsight, and try to climb them one after another without resting. A good grade to aim for should be 65 to 70 percent of your max, so V5 if you've redpointed V7. You should be trying hard, but the problems shouldn't be so hard that you're falling repeatedly. Climb the same problems without resting three more times (four times total), resting only a few minutes between rounds. As you get progressively more tired going through the rounds, your body should be more accustomed to every move and be able to do each problem more efficiently.

Keep It Short

True power training is very intense, only 45 to 60 minutes. Add in 15 to 30 minutes of warm-up and cooldown, and you're still done in less than two hours. By keeping these sessions short (fatigue creates endurance, not power), you can do more per week. If you're in decent shape, you can do up to two or three hard power sessions, totaling close to three hours of quality work. Typically, you want to focus on training power for no more than four to six weeks continuously. Any longer and you will stop seeing gains, or you might even get weaker. In a given year, you could fruitfully advance through three or four power phases. Intersperse these phases with, at minimum, four to six weeks of less-intense training or just climbing for fun.

Recovery Time Is Key

We don't leave the gym with more power—it's recovery that promotes improvement. In general, it should take thirty-six to seventy-two hours to bounce back from a proper power session. After this, it's critical that you again hit the system with another stimulus, or the first session's value declines. That means if you climb only once weekly, you'll see no improvement. On the flip side, rest too little or train too long (e.g., those fun four hours of nonstop gym routes with your buddies), and you fail to improve.

Specify

Specificity has two components. First, the more your training resembles your goal routes or problems, the better. Second, developing climbing power is about training the muscles of the back and the hip girdle. Sure, our arms get tired first, but it's these "big" muscles that generate the most force and help us integrate our feet and legs.

Don't Get Worked

At first, you might feel you aren't properly fatigued after a single session. Perfect! This lets you come back hard in a couple days. Improvement is why you're training. Be patient and be disciplined, and you'll see gains in as little as three weeks.

Speed It Up

Another good way to increase power is to increase speed. Because climbing is so technical, speed often decreases fine motor skill, hence accuracy when grabbing small holds. Only go a little bit faster at a time—say 5 percent—to prevent your form from going to hell. As an exercise, time yourself on some problems with ten to twelve moves; then speed them up by no more than a second or two. Work on efficiency. If you get sloppy, slow down and reevaluate.

A few tricks: Memorize the sequence from the ground, and climb from memory, not reaction. Move consistently upward: Don't start then stop, then start again. Instead, keep moving at a consistent pace. Focus on your feet; your legs drive most movement, so make sure they're not dragging behind you.

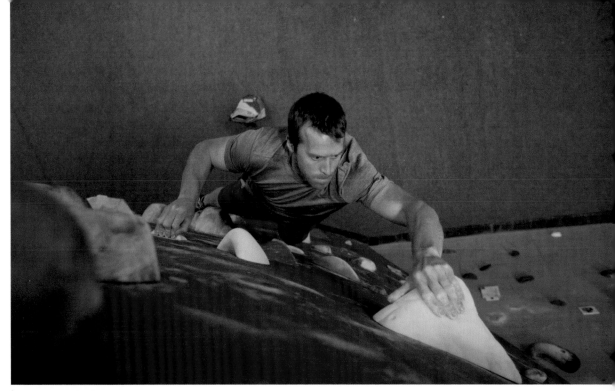
▶ *Tales of Power*

TALES OF POWER

You can train long or you can train hard, but not both, which is probably why so many of us train for power incorrectly. By "power," we mean the product of strength and speed, i.e., the explosive force recruited any time you use momentum, or "go for it." Properly training power allows you to get stronger, meaning pull harder and faster to get through otherwise impossible cruxes and do bigger moves. Step one with power training is to realize you're training, not just exercising. That means if you're still able to climb a steep wall on small holds three hours into a session, you're nowhere near your maximum ability and you're not really training power.

The Workout

This four-step workout looks almost too simple on paper, but it works. Try it a few days a week for three or four weeks, then test gains on personal benchmark problems.

> ▶ Fifteen to thirty minutes of warm-up, with resistance exercises (pull-ups and body weight squats) and some easier, yet increasingly intense, climbing. Cardiovascular exercise—a few minutes on the treadmill or stationary bike—is fine early in the warm-up, too.

▶ Four to five tries on a hard problem (four to ten moves), just above your onsight level, that requires explosive movement. Use holds big enough to train power, rather than failing because of finger strength. Think slopers, jugs, and big edges. If you don't quite top out, that's fine. Better to fail than to understimulate your system.

▶ Six to eight tries on one or two max-effort problems requiring explosiveness, with two to three minutes of rest between each burn. Again, if you complete more than half the problem, it's an attempt; though if you fall low, jump right back on. Remember, you are *not* going for a pump. If you feel fatigue, increase rest time. End this step when power declines even slightly.

▶ Cool down on easy ground, with stretching or exercises that recruit the opposite muscles of those you just worked, also called antagonist muscles. Because you've most likely been doing a lot of pulling, focus on pushing exercises: push-ups, bench dips, and some planks/bridges, with two to three sets of ten to twelve reps each, not quite to failure. This means you should be able to complete all the reps, but the final few reps should feel very difficult.

CREATE A CRUX

If you find yourself bored with the gym's set bouldering problems, you can make up dozens of new problems of your own with the holds already on the wall. When you create your own problems, you have limitless opportunities, and you're free to practice whatever weaknesses you have. You'll also push yourself mentally to be more creative during the problem-solving process, which can help you find better, more efficient ways to move through cruxes. Though there's no set training plan—you can do this whenever you want, at any difficulty level—the few suggestions below can help you spice up your gym time.

The Workout

▶ Find a group of friends to create problems with you. Having others around with fresh perspectives might challenge you in a way you didn't even know you needed help with. Don't complain if one of your partners chooses a powerful line up a steep wall that doesn't suit your techy, vertical skills; you might not ace the problem, but you'll gain valuable lessons while addressing your weak points.

▶ Take time to warm up. Spend the first half hour or more on easier problems. Start at V0, and slowly work your way up through the grades. Don't rush the process, and don't be afraid to repeat some harder color-coded problems put up by the gym's routesetters before you start the workout.

▶ Keep limits in mind. Take turns creating problems. Select a wall that inspires you, and make moves that do the same. In the beginning, it will be harder to create problems that aren't either too easy or overly hard. With time, you should be able to strike a balance, making problems that are one to four grades below your maximum redpoint ability. The idea isn't to project them for your entire climbing session; instead try a variety of problems on different walls.

▶ Project efficiently. The best method when trying harder problems is to give a good flash attempt, but if you fall, start again from the hold that kicked you off— not from the bottom. Trying the moves in isolation helps you piece the project together instead of wearing yourself out on the beginning and cutting your session short.

▶ Let there be a winner. Whoever climbs the problem first from bottom to top without falling gets to make up the next one.

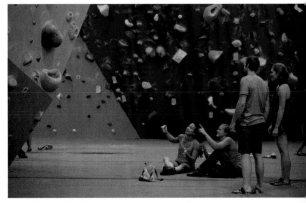

▶ *The more the merrier with Create a Crux.*

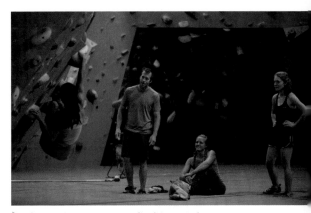

▶ *Incorporate many climbing styles.*

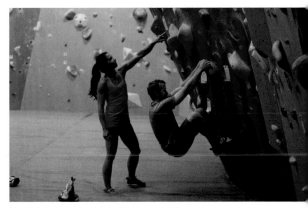

▶ *Help each other figure out beta.*

Tips to Create Better Problems

▶ Leave out the circus tricks. Create a problem that is relatively straightforward, with minimal feet and comfortable holds that have little chance of causing injury.

▶ Switch it up constantly. Don't get too attached to one problem or another.

▶ Don't make it easy. Try to create individual moves that you might not flash, but that you can do in a couple of tries. If you have a problem with four to six moves like that, then it's probably one to four grades below your max.

▶ Don't be scared to fail. Finding a move that may not be possible for you is one of the most interesting ideas in climbing. Think about progressing through a hard move like this: If you can touch a hold, you can grab it, and if you can grab it, then you can crank off it.

Keep moving around the gym, trying different combos on different walls. The variety will challenge all your muscle groups and technical skills, and give you a bigger bag of tricks to pull from.

▶ Take it seriously. Approach made-up lines just like any taped route in the gym, and even come back later in the session to repeat particularly hard or interesting problems. If you struggle on a certain project and can't top out before your crew moves on, make it a point to go back and work on that problem later, to address the weak spot it exposed.

▶ Know when to quit. If you regularly climb V7 and suddenly have trouble on V3s and V4s, your session might be over. However, because there's no specific grade attached to the problems you're creating, and therefore no real benchmark in difficulty, it can be hard to tell how rapidly your session is ending. One simple, direct method is to call it quits if you start to regress on moves that didn't feel too bad earlier in the session.

4X4'S AND CIRCUITS

Sometimes it's not the individual moves on a climb that are difficult, but rather linking them together. Enter power-endurance, or the ability to do multiple hard moves in a row. Train power-endurance with 4x4s or circuits so that difficult, pumpy sequences become easier. Training power-endurance forces your muscles to adapt and become better at creating adenosine triphosphate (ATP), which is the body's way to store and transport energy and helps release contracted muscle fibers when there's little to no oxygen available. It's essentially exposure therapy—you'll routinely bathe your forearms in lactic acid, and they'll respond by storing more energy in the cells to create ATP.

Power-endurance training is best done after establishing a solid base of strength and power training, because it will convert some of that maximum strength into endurance, and it can be excellent to focus on if you've been plateaued at the same

Game: Golf

Number of Players

2+

Setup

Pick six or more marked boulder problems or routes that are well within the players' ability levels; it helps to play against people who are of similar height and skill level. Each problem or route represents a "hole" on the hypothetical golf course.

How to Play

Players take turns trying to do each route or problem with as few holds as possible, and each player gets one go at the problem for each round. Each handhold used translates to a stroke. Each fall receives a three-stroke penalty. Keep track of each climber's score throughout. Whoever has the least amount of points at the end of the course wins.

Training Purpose

Route-finding, dynamic and deadpoint movement, power-endurance

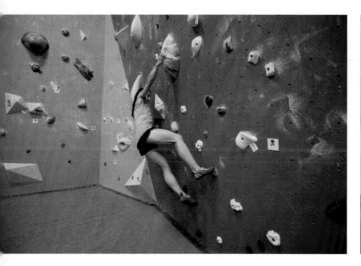
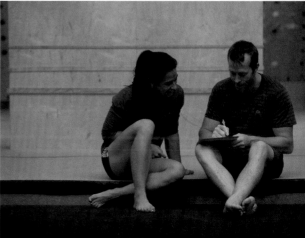

grade for a while. The common methods for training power-endurance involve lots of climbing, usually in circuits or 4x4s.

The Workout

Warm up by climbing easy terrain for about fifteen minutes. For the 4x4s, your muscles must be working hard, but not at their max, so focus on 50 to 80 percent of your limit. Power-endurance should make your forearms sore. Get forty-eight to seventy-two hours of rest between workouts. Start with two per week, and progress to three as soreness allows. You'll see gains in as little as two to three weeks, but you'll also lose those gains in about as much time. If you're not actively training, consider a power-endurance workout every couple of weeks to maintain your current level.

▶ **4x4s**: To complete a 4x4, pick four different boulder problems about three grades below your limit. Climb the first problem four times, dropping off and repeating the problem immediately, or downclimbing an easy route back to the start. Rest for two minutes, then climb the next problem the same way. Complete all four problems like this, then rest for five minutes. That's one set. Pick new problems, or repeat the same set again. Aim for three sets.

▶ **Circuits:** Pick three to five boulder problems, each three grades below your limit. Instead of climbing the same problem back-to-back, climb each problem once, only coming off the wall to move between them. This is your circuit. Your circuits can have rests, but don't remove your pump completely. After climbing your circuit once, rest for the same duration of time you spent on the wall. If you fall from being pumped, end your circuit and rest. If a foot slip or botched move spits you off, jump right back on. After completing your circuit four times with equal-length rests, take a longer break of five to ten minutes. Next, start another set of four circuits on the same or new problems. Mimic your project if you have one. For example, if it's a long section of V1 followed by a V3 at the top, pick three problems in the V1 range, followed by a V3. You'll progress in your circuits by either shortening your rests or by choosing harder problems. Try starting sets thirty seconds sooner, and see how much harder the problems feel.

LIMIT BOULDERING

Climbing a lot is great for your overall fitness, but after you've reached a baseline strength, you won't see improvements on the climbing wall unless you try things at or above your personal limit. Many problems set in the bouldering gym only have a handful of difficult moves, and those moves might be separated by large holds or rests. With limit bouldering, you create your own mini sequences so that you're doing a few really hard moves in a row. The biggest benefit here is that you can train hard, technical movement while also training power. Though the concept is simple, it's important to stick to the exercise and not get distracted trying to send preset gym problems.

The Workout

Warm up by climbing easy terrain for about fifteen minutes, focusing on getting your shoulders primed to do hard moves. Large and small shoulder circles (both directions) or working with a TheraBand can focus in on those small stabilizing muscles of the shoulder. (Check out page 123 for simple shoulder routines.) Find several boulder sequences that are near your personal limit. There should be only three to seven hard moves—none of the moves should be easy. The goal is to do repeated powerful movements that force deadpointing (grabbing a hold at the apex of a movement) and sticking difficult holds. Make up a sequence (you don't have to stick

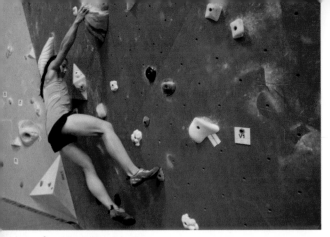

▶ *Limit Bouldering*

to the established problems), and give it a go. If you complete it on the first try, it's too easy. If you fall off the first move, consider that one attempt. Rest two to three minutes before trying again, focusing on form, power, and precision. After you've given this sequence three to five solid attempts, move on to another and repeat the process.

Try four to five different sequences, aiming to climb thirty minutes to an hour. Rest more if you don't feel fresh between attempts, and stop as soon as you feel fatigued. You may feel like you're not climbing enough, but power is being trained even though you won't feel trashed. Throw an hour of limit bouldering into your routine once or twice a week, and keep a few sequences as benchmarks so that when you try them week after week, you can see noticeable improvements.

MOONBOARD

Created by British climber Ben Moon in 2005, the MoonBoard is a standardized bouldering wall with identical holds placed in the same orientation in a grid pattern. The idea is that all MoonBoards across the world match, so everyone who has access to one can climb the same problems. Originally Moon created a downloadable list of problems that could be printed out, but now there's an app that lets you

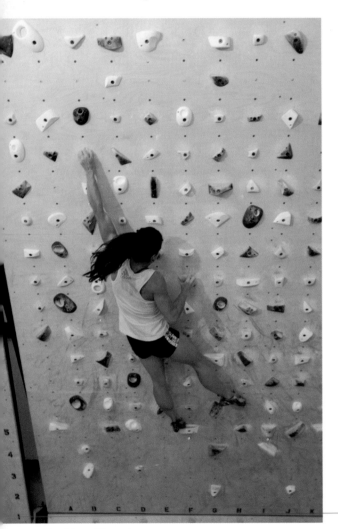

▶ *MoonBoard*

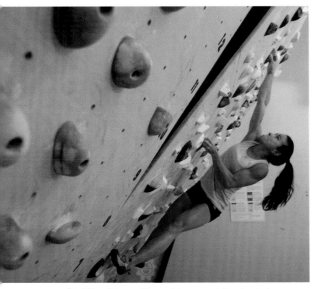

▶ *The MoonBoard is great for training strength and power.*

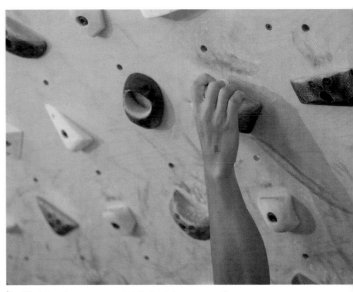

▶ *Lights show you which holds are on for a particular problem.*

access a database of every problem on your phone—and add your own. Tracking your progress and comparing beta with climbers all over the world, whether they're average Joes or pros, is a really fun way to stay motivated. With MoonBoards regaining popularity in the last few years, many gyms have them, so ask at the front desk if one is available.

The Workout

There's no specific way to use the MoonBoard, but it's really fun and addictive, especially if you do it with friends. You can do as much or as little as you want in any given day, and it can be a nice break from serious training. The steep angle and challenging holds build power, strengthen the core, and improve finger strength. Consider working in one session per week, or a few per month. The holds are infamously difficult to cling to, so make sure to warm up well on easier problems in the bouldering area before trying anything too difficult. Don't be discouraged if you can't send any of the problems in the beginning. The beauty of the MoonBoard is that the holds and wall don't change that often, so you can use certain problems or moves to monitor your overall strength and progress as a climber.

SAMPLE TRAINING WEEK

If you've been climbing for a little while and want to start dabbling in focused training, following an organized weekly program is a great next step. Any type of fitness training centers on consistency. You can do almost anything when you go to the gym, and if you stick with it long enough, you'll see results. Going to the gym randomly and climbing around is great in the beginning, but it's hard to measure your progress. Committing to a detailed multi-month program can be overwhelming. This sample training week strikes a nice balance between the two, making structured training much more manageable. It offers some direction for what to do in the gym on any given day of the week, but you don't have to commit to anything complicated.

The Workout

Following is a daily breakdown of a sample training week. This sample starts on Monday, as a rest day, assuming you climbed or were active over the weekend. However, you can, of course, start on whichever day works best for you and adjust rest/training days as necessary to fit your schedule. If you relaxed over the weekend, consider bumping all the training up a day so you're working out on Monday. Using the following Sample Training Week, build a 4-week plan that dials up the intensity each week based on how you're feeling. So if certain holds on the hangboard feel easier in Week 2 than Week 1, consider using smaller holds for Weeks 3 and 4. The same goes for the weighted exercises and the climbing—try heavier weights (only add a few pounds at a time) and harder problems for on-the-wall sessions. Stick to your program for 4 weeks, take a week off and just do easy climbing for fun, and then come back to your climbing projects and see how they feel. If you're feeling stronger, create another 4- or 6-week program. You can do as many programs as you want in a year. Just make sure to take 1 to 2 weeks off in between sets to let your body recover and maximize the benefits. Take more rest time if the program was high intensity.

MONDAY

EXERCISE	SETS	REPS	REST
REST DAY			

TUESDAY

EXERCISE	SETS	REPS	REST

WARM UP

Bouldering: 6–8 problems; 3 minutes rest between each

HANGBOARDING

10 seconds on / 10 seconds off (x3, any holds), 4–10 sets, rest 4 minutes between each

TRX SHOULDER STRENGTHENING

TRX reverse flys, TRX Ys, and TRX Is; 15 reps each per set; 3–6 sets; rest 1 minute between each

TRX CORE ROUTINE

TRX plank, TRX reverse crunches, TRX mountain climbers, TRX plank (again), TRX oblique crunches;
1 minute each

WEDNESDAY

EXERCISE	SETS	REPS	REST

WARM-UP

Bouldering: 6–8 problems; 3 minutes rest between each

PROJECTING

Project 2–6 boulder problems; rest 10 minutes between each

SHOULDER FITNESS

Dumbbell shoulder presses, dumbbell lateral raises, dumbbell reverse flies, dumbbell front raises;
12 reps each per set; 3–6 sets, rest 1 minute between each

SHOULDER RECOVERY ROUTINE

Band external rotation, band elevated external rotation, band internal rotation, lying dumbbell external
rotation; 20 reps each; 2 sets; no rest between

THURSDAY

EXERCISE	SETS	REPS	REST
REST DAY			

FRIDAY

EXERCISE	SETS	REPS	REST

WARM-UP

Bouldering: 6–8 problems; 3 minutes rest between each

BACK AND BICEPS ROUTINE

Barbell bent-over rows, dumbbell bent-over rows, dumbbell bicep curls, dumbbell hammer curls, pull-ups; 12 reps each; 2–5 sets; rest 1 minute between each set

SHOULDER RECOVERY ROUTINE

Band external rotation, band elevated external rotation, band internal rotation, lying dumbbell external rotation; 20 reps each; 2 sets; no rest between

SATURDAY

EXERCISE	SETS	REPS	REST

WARM-UP

Route climbing; 4–6 routes; 8 minutes rest between each

HARD/EASY/HARD

Climb a hard route, then an easy route, then a hard route consecutively; 3–6 sets; 15 minutes rest between each set

TRX SIDE PLANKS

Hold one minute on each side; 3–5 sets; 1 min. rest between each set

SUNDAY

EXERCISE	SETS	REPS	REST

CLIMB WHATEVER YOU WANT!

This day is up to you. Have fun!

SHOULDER RECOVERY ROUTINE

Band external rotation, band elevated external rotation, band internal rotation, lying dumbbell external rotation; 20 reps each; 2 sets; no rest between

BOULDER THREE GRADES HARDER IN ONE YEAR

Being motivated and dedicated is the key to reaching any goal. This year-long program, geared toward intermediate and advanced climbers, will help you get stronger and more powerful, but you have to work for it. Try this program, which requires a full year of commitment, if you've been climbing for a while and have plateaued at a certain grade. Training like this is all about consistency and dedication, but you will have success if you keep at it. If you're doing any other training program, make sure to have at least two weeks of light climbing or active rest before start-

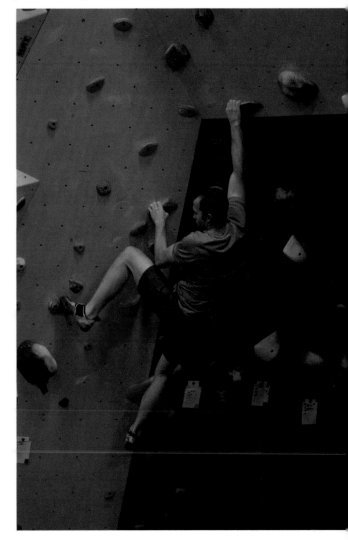

ing this. "Trying hard" is being so tired you have to crawl across the bouldering pads to your next problem, having determination to succeed, and refusing to stop or give up. This is how you need to approach your training. Hard work beats talent when talent stops working hard, so bottom line is: Work hard!

That said, be careful not to burn out. Training is very demanding. If you are extremely tired during training, are unmotivated, and/or are not improving, take a break. Just climb for fun.

For each day, do a dynamic warm-up for fifteen minutes with jumping jacks, leg kicks, shoulder circles, push-ups, etc. Boulder on easy problems for ten more minutes, then begin your program. This schedule is based on training Monday through Friday, and climbing or resting on weekends. The following program has acronyms for many of the exercises. See the Exercise Key on the following pages for explanations of each exercise.

MONTH 1: POWER

Power is the explosive strength that sets bouldering apart from other types of climbing. If you want to boulder hard, you need to build power.

CLIMB: CLM, CB, CLAD, CTD, 4x4, SPU (see Exercise Key on page 66)

CROSS: Core

MONTH 2: STRENGTH

This month boosts your ability to hold onto and move off difficult holds in any direction.

CLIMB: As many hard problems as you can per session; WPU, SPU

PINCH HANGS: Straight-arm hang on two pinches on the system board (TF)

PINCH PULL-UPS: Pull-ups on those same pinches on the system board (TF)

PAD-CRIMP PULL-UPS: Use a rung on the campus board that you can put a full finger pad on (TF)

FRENCHIES: Do a pull-up and go side to side (TF), then rest 90 seconds between sets

CROSS: Core; push-ups (TF)

MONTH 3: POWER-ENDURANCE

Now you'll work on power-endurance—your capacity to do multiple hard moves in a row with intensity, accuracy, and power.

CLIMB: Pyramids: 8-6-4-4-6-8. Choose a grade for each set. (A V5 climber would start around V2.) For example: 8 V2s, 6 V3s, 4 V4s, 4 V4s, 6 V3s, 8 V2s. After each problem up the pyramid, do 10 push-ups. On the way down the pyramid, do 5 pull-ups after each problem.

CROSS: Core; running (30- to 45-minute jog)

MONTH 4: POWER

Repeat Month 1, but you should be able to complete harder throws, use smaller rungs, and increase grades for 4x4s.

CLIMB: CLM, CB, CLAD, CTD, 4x4, SPU

CROSS: Core

MONTH 5: PROJECTING

Time to try boulders above your limit. If you feel a decrease in power, you can add a campus day once a week.

CLIMB: See how you have progressed by projecting boulder problems.

CROSS: Core

MONTH 6: POWER AND CROSS-TRAINING

Time to build superior general fitness with more cross-training.

CLIMB: CLM, CB, CLAD, CTD, 4x4, SPU

CROSS: Core; circuits: push-ups, pull-ups, dumbbell shoulder presses, ring push-ups, bent-over rows, wide push-ups, biceps curls, burpees, mountain climbers, pull-up lockoffs. Each exercise is 45 seconds; don't rest until you complete the circuit. After completing one round, rest for 2 minutes and repeat 5 times. Pick a weight that is pushing your limit at the end of 45 seconds.

MONTH 7: ENDURANCE

Boulder problems require endurance, too. The key to increasing yours? Getting on longer routes, which is a welcome change of pace.

CLIMB:

1 hard route twice; rest 5 minutes; 6 sets
5 routes (2 hard, 2 medium, 1 easy); 1 set
3 problems that go up in grade; rest 3 minutes; 3 sets
5 boulder problems (2 hard, 2 medium, 1 easy); rest 5 minutes; 2 sets

CROSS: Pull-ups (TF), then push-ups (TF); rest 90 seconds; 5 sets

MONTH 8: SYSTEM BOARD

Overcome weaknesses with targeted movements; do everything on the same days or alternate.

CLIMB: Simulate difficult moves and focus on weaknesses (body positions, bad holds, etc.). After an hour and a half of this, climb and project for fun.

CROSS: Core; any cross-training (running, cycling, circuits, etc.)

MONTH 9: FINGER STRENGTH

Climb 3 to 4 days a week; make sure to take at least one full rest day a week.

CLIMB: Double-arm lockoff on campus rungs; pull up and hold for 10 seconds, then 5 seconds off. Repeat 5 times for one set, rest for 3 minutes, 6 sets. Halfway lockoff: Same sequence as full lockoff, except arms should be bent at 90 degrees. Deadhang: Same sequence as lockoffs, but let your arms hang straight. Climb every problem of your onsight grade in the bouldering area in 1 hour.

CROSS: Run

MONTH 10: POWER

Repeat Months 1 and 4, but increase difficulty of each exercise. Project difficult problems inside.

CLIMB: CLM, CB, CGOA, CDC, CLMB; project hard climbs

CROSS: Core

MONTH 11: POWER-ENDURANCE

Focus on climbing-specific exercises to prepare for projecting.

CLIMB: CLAD (4 sets), 4x4

PINCH PULL-UPS: 10 reps per set; 10 sets; rest 2 minutes between sets

PINCH LOCKOFFS: 10–30 seconds per set; 10 sets; rest 2 minutes between sets

4X4 (AGAIN): Do one 4x4 with one moderate problem (last exercise for the session)

CROSS: None

MONTH 12: CRUSH!

Projecting boulder problems is three parts creativity, five parts persistence, and seven parts patience. Don't be upset when you fail one, two, or ten times. Working through movements at our physical and mental limits can be the most exhausting thing in the world. But by failing repeatedly, we are forced to utilize the more abstract levels of our minds to come up with a solution. It might mean that "Eureka!" moment, or stumbling upon beta that seems crazy at first but finally makes your project possible. Don't rule anything out when you're projecting, and think outside the box. Being patient with and committed to the process of overcoming failure is the only way to the top of any problem.

*Each exercise comprises 6 sets with a 2-minute rest between each set, unless otherwise noted.

**All campus moves start matched on the same rung, with feet on small foot rungs if needed.

***TF = to failure

Exercise Key

Below are explanations of each exercise listed in the Boulder Three Grades Harder program. Some exercises are very specific (e.g., Campus Long Move), while others can be interpreted with more flexibility (e.g., Core).

4x4

Repeat one moderately difficult boulder problem 4 times, rest 4 minutes, then pick a new problem and repeat it 4 times, until you've done a total of 4 sets. By the fourth go on each problem, you should be trying hard to finish.

Campus Bumps (CB)

Move one hand up each rung as high as you can reach, and then bump back down each rung to your starting position. Go immediately up with the opposite hand; climb at least three to four rungs.

Campus Double-Clutch (CDC)

Start matched on a rung, throw with both hands to the next rung, and try to campus back down to the beginning rung. Go to failure for one set.

Campus Go-Again (CGOA)

Start matched on one rung, throw up to a rung, and come back down to the matched position, then do it again immediately with the same arm. One set is completing three throws on each side.

Campus Ladder (CLAD)

Climb like a ladder, with each hand going above the other (you can skip rungs or match hands as needed). Match at the top, then downclimb to the beginning and immediately go again—complete as many ladders as you can in one set without rest.

Campus Long Move, Bump Back Down (CLMB)

Do the campus long move, then bump directly back down to the starting rung. Do each side once for one set.

Campus Long Move (CLM)

Throw with one arm to the highest rung you can reach. Come off the board and immediately repeat the same movement with the other arm. Each side is one set.

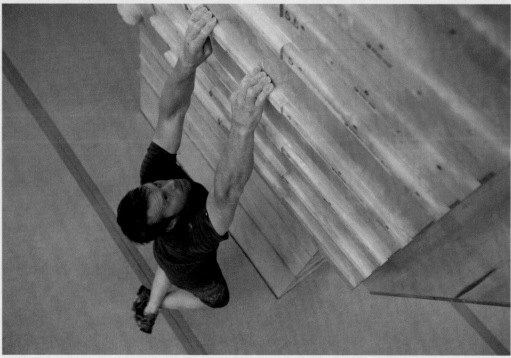
▶ *Deadhang on Campus Rungs*

Campus Touch/Drop (CTD)

Throw up to max level, latch the rung, and come back to match hands without coming off. Complete three reps on each arm before touching the ground.

Core

Do any combination of core exercises, but rest a minute or two after each exercise, then repeat for a total 20- to 25-minute core session. Options: toes to bar, front levers (2 minutes), planks (2 minutes), V-ups, Russian twists (1 minute), sit-ups (2 minutes).

Speed Pull-Up (SPU)

Do a pull-up quickly, lower slowly, then go right back up. Go to failure for each set.

Weighted Pull-Up (WPU)

Add enough weight when doing pull-ups to ensure that your second to fourth pull-ups are hard; two to four reps per set.

Game: Add-On

Number of Players

2+ (smaller groups work better)

Setup

Pick a sequence of three or four moves that all the players can do, and then decide who goes first.

How to Play

The first climber does the predetermined sequence, adding one "move," typically defined as one hand movement with set footholds (foot movements are not considered standalone moves). The next climber repeats the new sequence and adds a move of his own. If a climber cannot perform the previously added sequence, he loses a life. If he completes the added-on move, this is considered a checkpoint. Even if he fails to add another move, he is safe. Three failed attempts (lives lost) means elimination. Continue adding on moves until (1) you're all bored; (2) you run out of room and don't feel like traversing; or (3) one climber is left standing. It's optional if you want to let other players help the climber remember the sequence by pointing out holds.

Training Purpose

Route-finding, memorizing sequences, endurance, working on weaknesses (especially when playing with someone who climbs differently than you—tall versus short, crimp versus compression, etc.)

Add-On Variations

5 Seconds: Right before you latch any hold you're about to add, hover your hand over it for a full five seconds.

Feet Only: Switch it so feet are the focus and add foot moves; all hands are on.

Bonus: If you can skip any previous move, you can "steal" that move and add an extra move at the end of your regular turn (e.g., skip one move, add two at the end).

Directional: Go one direction the first round; go the opposite direction the next round, still adding moves if you can.

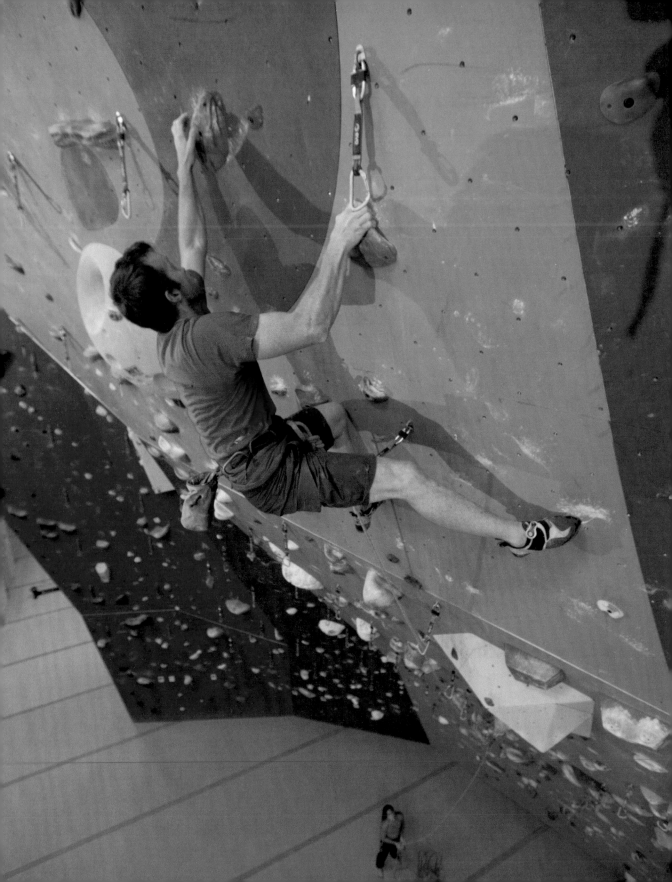

Chapter 3

ENDURANCE

AS IN ALL OTHER ATHLETIC ENDEAVORS, climbing endurance translates to the ability to sustain effort over a period of time. That means holding onto the wall and moving upward for more than just a few minutes; elite athletes can climb without coming off for a few hours. Other sports reference endurance in terms of cardio fitness, but in climbing, it's more about "local endurance," meaning a certain muscle group's ability to sustain effort over time. So what's the most important muscle group for climbers? The forearms.

Of course climbers use every muscle group, but the forearms are usually the least developed, especially when you're first starting out. While you train forearm endurance, you'll also increase endurance for the rest of your body, including cardio, legs, and core. Roped routes are longer and require more endurance to complete, so the following workouts focus primarily on roped climbing. Endurance is factored into the grade of roped routes, meaning individual moves are usually easier than those found in bouldering, there are bigger holds, and there are spots where you can rest and get some energy back. Resting on-route is a huge part of sending roped routes, so that is a key component of endurance training.

Figuring out the sequences on a roped climb is a fun and engaging process, but it's much less social than bouldering because you are either climbing on the wall or belaying your partner. One thing to keep in mind is that training endurance primarily helps you with climbing longer routes (as opposed to training strength, which helps with all types of climbing). If you enjoy roped climbing, consider focusing on endurance and strength equally, splitting your time between the two. If you want to get a full-body strength workout with the added benefit of some aerobic training, or you just prefer to be on the wall for longer periods, consider the following endurance workouts.

CLIMB FOREVER WITH ARC SETS

When climbing, your forearms fail because blood isn't getting to the muscle tissue. But it's not because your heart isn't working fast enough: Instead, the blood has trouble reaching your forearms because the muscle fibers have locked up, along with the blood vessels. The most popular form of local endurance training for climbers is called ARC training, which stands for Aerobic, Respiration, and Capillarity. The aim of ARC training is to increase the number of the tiny blood vessels (capillaries) in your forearms. By climbing lots of terrain below your limit, you'll actually develop more small blood vessels, and the existing ones will become wider. Both changes make it harder for a pump to set in, meaning you can climb longer and recover faster.

The Workout

ARC training is done by climbing easy terrain for fifteen to forty-five minutes at a time while maintaining a very light pump. Two common methods include traversing a bouldering wall, or moving up and down routes on toprope or autobelay without coming off.

First, pick a type of terrain to cover, like slab, vertical, or steep. Vertical to slightly overhanging terrain is best because it keeps some weight on your arms, but not too much. It's better to find a route or section of the wall with multiple angles in this range. Training on different angles allows you to fine-tune your technique, and helps break up the monotony of long sets.

Next, figure out how hard your target route or traverse should be. If you've never done ARC-style training before, start at 5.6 or 5.7 and up the grade as necessary. If you're traversing or don't have a graded route to climb, use holds that create a light pump that you can maintain for a long time.

The climbing should be fairly continuous, with no hard moves that could cause you to fall. It's best if you can move without pausing to shake out frequently. The idea is to be climbing and moving for as long as possible. For a first-timer, regardless of redpoint ability, moving continuously on the wall for ten minutes might feel

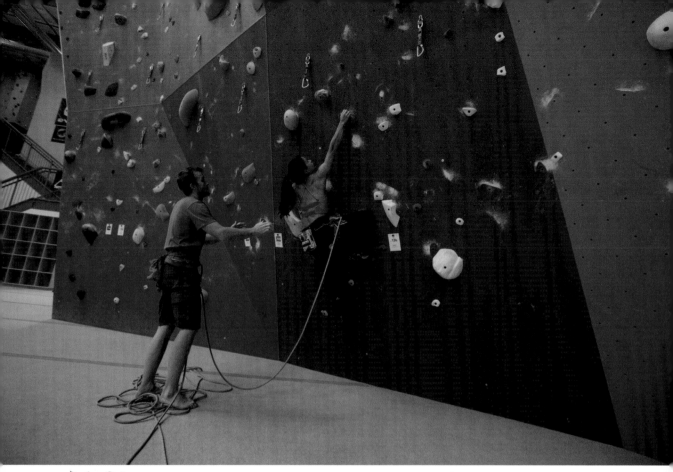

▶ *Arc Sets*

impossible, even on a vertical 5.6 or V0 boulder problem. If this happens to you, try sets of 5 minutes on, 5 minutes off, aiming for a total on-the-wall time of 30 to 45 minutes per session. Next session, try 10 minutes on, 10 minutes off, and so on. Advanced climbers may need to start just as low as beginners if they've never done local endurance training, but all climbers should progress quickly.

As for scheduling, do two to four ARC sets in each week of ARC training (up to about four weeks), or mix in one session per week with other training. ARC training is very low intensity, so it can be done often without stressing your muscles and joints. In fact, ARC training can be a good way to actively recover the day after a harder workout. Next time you take extended time off from climbing, do a couple of weeks of local endurance training to ease back into it. It'll work technique and establish a good baseline you can build from.

Mix it Up

ARC training is one of the best ways to train local endurance, but it can be boring to stay on the wall, pulling easy move after easy move, for half an hour. Mix up your ARC routine by trying out these ideas:

▶ Do technique drills (see page 39). Pick a technique, like kneebars, and do as many as possible for five minutes. Pick another technique, like flagging, for the next five minutes. Work these techniques while downclimbing, too.

▶ Focus on body position. Can you bring your hips in more or rotate them differently? Do you need both feet on for that move? Could you use a lower foot and cross through instead?

▶ Find as many ways as possible to get from one hold to the next—which was best and why?

▶ Focus on your breathing. Keep a steady breathing pattern, but mix in a harder move or two every few minutes with strong, focused exhales.

▶ Get ARC benefits by climbing with a partner, or by mimicking ARC-style training outside. Any exercise that focuses on the volume, and not the difficulty, of climbing helps.

▶ Try to climb every boulder in the gym that's at or below a certain grade, like V1 or V0, taking short rests between problems to avoid getting pumped. Climb up and then downclimb for extra mileage, resting when needed. You won't gain ARC benefits if you become too pumped, but the more continuous time you spend on the wall, the better. Or climb all the toprope routes in the gym that feel moderate and don't pump you out. Alternate routes in your local gym with a partner, only stopping to switch belays between routes.

▶ Grab a partner and climb pitches at least a grade below your onsight level. Try to climb two to three pitches at a time back to back, then switch with your partner. Aim for at least ten pitches. You shouldn't feel a strong pump at any point. Drop a grade or two if you do, especially toward the end of a session. Think of it as a slightly more intense, all-day warm-up, after which you go home.

▶ You can use one round of a shorter ARC session as a warm-up for any climbing or training session.

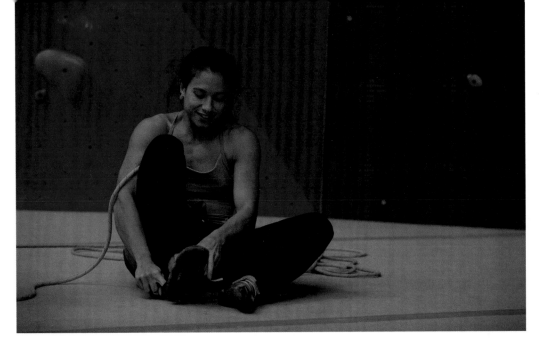

LEAPFROG

This is a creative take on endurance training for climbers of all ability levels. The basic idea is to climb, downclimb, and reclimb the same sections of terrain so you are on the same route for a longer period of time. Because it includes downclimbing, your technique also improves as you learn the holds and nuances of each move, and because it includes reclimbing, you'll become more efficient at all the moves. Keep in mind that you'll need an attentive belay that lasts a while, so make sure your partner is willing to help out. Be willing to offer the same long belay! This drill can be adapted for shorter amounts of time, but a full session could take up to two hours, including rest time.

The Workout

Pick a route at least two grades below your onsight level. This includes + and - ratings; for example, if you onsight 5.11-, find a 5.10 for this drill. If your gym grades using letters, pick a route that is two or three letters below your onsight level; for example, if you onsight 5.11a, find a 5.10c or b. If the first rep of the drill feels overly difficult, pick an easier route so you can complete multiple reps of the Leapfrog.

Start by climbing the beginning of the route, clipping the first three quickdraws, as usual. Once you have made the third clip, begin to downclimb. Downclimb to the clipping stance at the second quickdraw, being sure to mimic your previous body position at the clipping stance. Then, continue to climb upward to make the fourth clip. Once you have clipped the fourth draw, downclimb to the clipping stance at the third. From this stance, climb up to make your next clip.

Continue to the top of the route in this fashion; each time you make a clip, downclimb to the previous quickdraw, settle into the clipping stance, then again continue upward. Once you have clipped the anchors, you have finished one rep. You do not need to downclimb from the anchor. Switch with your partner, then repeat the drill on the same route. It is OK to fall while doing the Leapfrog—if you fall near the top, simply lower and count the attempt as one rep. After you have completed the route three times, take a fifteen-minute rest. Then, choose a new route and repeat the drill again. Aim for three more attempts on the new route.

If this feels too difficult, build up endurance with variations of the drill. Instead of downclimbing at each clip, try climbing the entire route, downclimbing to the midpoint, then climbing back up to the top. Once this is doable, build up to the complete Leapfrog.

TREADWALL TRAINING

Rotating climbing walls, the most common brand name being Treadwalls, are perfect if you want to train endurance but don't have a partner. Not all gyms have them, but if yours does, definitely try them out. They can offer solitude and focus in a crowded, noisy gym. Because you don't need to communicate with a partner or worry about people walking below you (as it is sectioned off from the rest of the gym), it's a great chance to wear headphones and listen to a podcast or playlist while you climb. Most Treadwalls have adjustable angles and speeds to make them steeper and more difficult. There are plenty of ways to use the Treadwall; read on for two approaches.

The Workouts

Mega-Enduro ARC Sets: Using the same Aerobic, Respiration, and Capillarity principles we explored earlier, you'll use this training to break through a plateau caused by insufficient endurance or the inability to recover properly on a route. An effective ARC workout involves pinpointing the level at which you can sustain climbing despite feeling a low-level pump—roughly three to four letter grades below your redpoint. Flamed forearms are not the goal. Start your timer and begin climbing.

Aim for three sets of 20 to 30 minutes each, though you can also do two 45-minute sessions. Sweating and heavier breathing after about 10 minutes indicate the right intensity, but you should never feel at risk of falling. Practice inhaling through the nose, then exhaling strongly through the mouth as you climb. Focus on efficient movement, and find counterintuitive rest positions, stems, high steps, and holds where you need to alternate hands. Find a jug on the side of the wall, within reach of the on/off switch for the wall, and shake out for a few seconds periodically,

Game: Eliminator

Number of Players

1+ (smaller groups work better, can be played alone)

Setup

Pick a route or boulder problem well within the players' ability—the more moves, the better.

How to Play

Climbers take turns repeating the problem; one person eliminates a hold after each successful round of attempts. If the next climber can't do the new sequence, it gets passed on to the next climber. When nobody is capable of doing the sequence, the climber who eliminated the hold must prove the sequence can be done. Keep going until either only one person or nobody can do the sequence.

Training Purpose

Creative route-finding, figuring out beta, dynamic and deadpoint movement without coming off. After each ARC session, rest on the ground as long as the time spent on the wall, or until the pump has subsided.

Intervals: This is ultra-high-intensity training, meaning you should barely be able to finish each set—going full anaerobic. Once you see improvements, increase the wall's angle or add a weight vest. For best results, complete this workout twice a week, with one or two days of rest between sessions. Map out a thirty-move route. Prerun the route to ensure the moves are at a high intensity relative to your ability— think hard flash or onsight.

Complete five sets, resting two minutes between each. If you can, monitor your heart rate during intervals, aiming to keep it at or below 90 percent of your max heart rate. (The average max heart rate for twenty-year-olds is 200 beats per minute [bpm], for thirty-year-olds 190 bpm, and for forty-year-olds 180 bpm.) Climb at a steady pace and in a precise manner. Focus on proper breathing, grabbing holds well, and precision hand and foot placement. This will translate to better performance on difficult projects later.

PYRAMIDS

Every climber's resume looks like a pyramid, where the bottom is a solid base of easier climbs and, as you go up, there are fewer hard climbs at the top. Getting better is all about mileage, so if you're having difficulty climbing harder grades, it's

Tips for Successful ARCing

▶ To up the ante, wear a weight vest. Start with just a few pounds. Add weight gradually, up to 15 percent of body weight. When that becomes too easy, change the hold sequence or steepness to add difficulty.

▶ For longer routes, number the holds in addition to having them color-coded or taped; doing so lets you "skip" holds on the fly, keeping you from gravitating toward the same sequences and helping prevent repetitive-use injuries.

▶ Keep a stopwatch or smartphone with a timing app handy. Use a fan to stay cool as the pump mounts.

always worthwhile to go back and climb more of the easier stuff. The wider your pyramid base is, the stronger your foundation and the easier it will be to add more ticks to the top.

The Workout

Pick a number grade you feel consistent with. If you're a solid 5.11 climber, then go with 5.10. Without untying from the rope or resting between attempts, climb 5.10a to 5.10d, then back down from 5.10d to 5.10a. If you fall below halfway up the route, start that route over and try to complete it, and then keep moving through the pyramid. If you fall again below halfway, move on to the next route. If you fall above the halfway point, count it and move on to the next route. By the end of the pyramid, you should have climbed eight routes without rests in between. Rest at least fifteen to twenty minutes, and then go another round. Advanced climbers can shoot for three rounds. Below are some examples of what a pyramid might look like.

5.11 roped climber: 5.10a, 5.10b, 5.10c, 5.10d, 5.10d, 5.10c, 5.10b, 5.10a

V8 boulderer: V4, V5, V6, V7, V7, V6, V5, V4

ROPED INTERVALS

Intervals are a secret training weapon for any sport. The idea is to follow a strict schedule of work and rest, so that you're trying really hard and then resting completely. One big benefit of interval training is that it's a very efficient way to train, meaning you get more bang for your buck in the gym. Another major benefit is that it helps burn more calories, both during the workout and afterward.

The Workout

Perform a series of difficult, four-minute climbing burns with only five minutes rest between each climb. You and your partner take turns climbing (toprope or lead) for four minutes, while the other belays. There's a one-minute transition period between each climb—be sure to double-check both the knot and belay device with each changeover. Select routes within two full number grades of your onsight limit—for example, if you onsight 5.10, then climb between 5.8 and 5.10. Use a stopwatch to stay on schedule. If you finish the route with time to spare, immediately begin downclimbing the route, stopping at the four-minute mark. When your four minutes are up, lower to the ground, untie, and belay your partner on his or her climb. Do at least six climbs each—this will take exactly one hour if you stay on schedule. Beginners should shoot for at least six climbs, while intermediate and advanced climbers should try to get at least twelve four-minute burns in.

VOLUME FOR POINTS

One of the best aspects of the climbing gym is the social and fun atmosphere. People are chatting, music is playing, and energy is high. The only problem is that

Why Do We Get Pumped?

Feeling pumped means the muscles in your arms aren't getting enough oxygen-rich blood, which helps muscles create the chemical ATP efficiently. ATP is required to release muscle fibers after they've been contracted, so if there isn't enough ATP available, your muscles can't relax. This is why you have a hard time opening and closing your hands when you're really pumped. Once muscle fibers lock up, they squeeze the tiny blood vessels (capillaries) in your forearms shut, which means less oxygen reaches other fibers as well, and the pump grows in a vicious cycle. When zero blood is reaching your muscles, the muscles seize up and you fall. The goal of local-endurance training is to prevent that shutdown of blood supply, providing your forearms with ATP so fibers can relax and flex with each move.

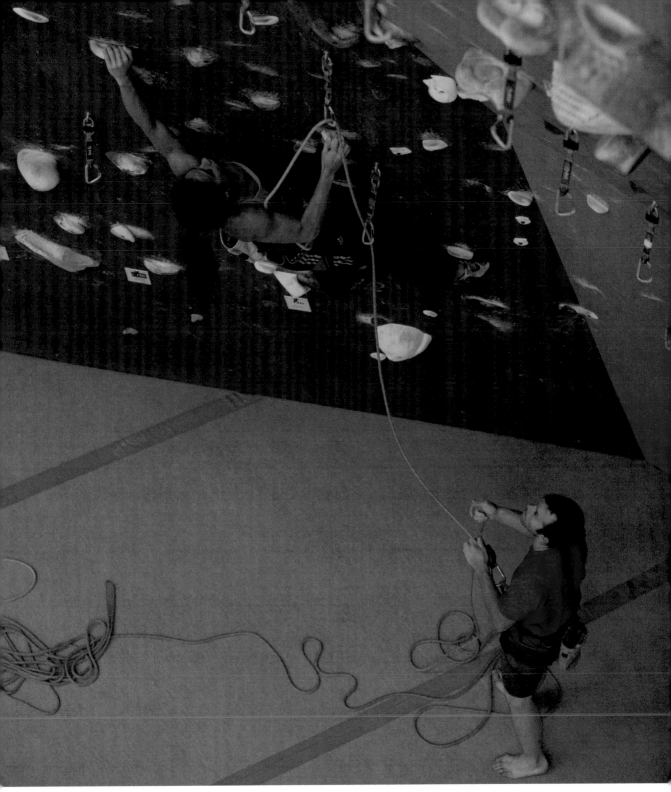

▶ *Roped Intervals*

those very elements can also distract from the task at hand—actually climbing. Volume for Points tracks how much you've climbed in a single session and ensures you've gotten a solid workout despite the distractions. The idea is simple: Each route or problem is worth a certain number of points; when you reach the top, add those points to your overall tally. You can customize this based on how much time you have, and you can do it on a rope, which will build more endurance, or in the bouldering area, which will build more strength.

The Workout

This is best done three times a week, with a day of rest between each session, for four weeks in a row. Focus on incremental progress for that month, followed by an easier fifth week, and then try your project. It's great for the end of a setting cycle, when the problems or routes have been up for a while and you have them wired. The climb's grade is the point value, but you get double points if the climb is at your onsight level. For example, a V6 boulderer gets five points for a V5, but twelve

GAME: Lemon–Lime

Number of Players

1

Setup

Pick a boulder problem that's doable but slightly challenging for you.

How to Play

Make the first move of the problem, and then reverse to the start. Without coming off, make the first two moves, and then go back to the start. Keep going until you've reached the top. That's the lemon! For the lime, do the same thing with downclimbing—without coming off. Start at the top, downclimb one move, then go back to the top. Two moves down, then back to the top. Once you've downclimbed to the start and back up to the top, you can jump off.

Training Purpose

Endurance, endurance, endurance—and power-endurance

points for a V6. Set a number goal and climb until you reach it, getting as much rest as you need within that session. Beginners set lower number goals, and intermediate/advanced climbers set higher point goals.

V6 boulderer (points/day)
Week 1: 40
Week 2: 45–50
Week 3: 50–55
Week 4: 55–60
5.10 sport climber (points/day)
Week 1: 100
Week 2: 150
Week 3: 200
Week 4: 250

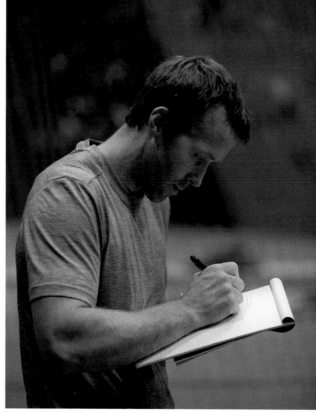

▶ *Keep a record of your Volume for Points training.*

LAPS

Laps are the climbing equivalent of running laps on a track, except way more fun and interesting because you're on a vertical climbing wall. They work local climbing endurance, but also put an emphasis on cardiovascular fitness. Perhaps the best part is that, if your gym has an autobelay, you can climb as many laps as you want without making your belayer suffer!

The Workout

Pick a grade range that clocks in around 70 percent of your max redpoint level. A 5.11+ climber should climb 5.10+ with a few 5.11- routes thrown in. Climb five routes in your range, with no rest between each. If the five routes feel impossible, then go to an easier grade or try four routes. Take a fifteen- to twenty-minute rest between sets, or belay your partner for a break. Repeat the set of five laps, trying different climbs. If there aren't enough routes in the range, it's OK to repeat. Beginners should aim for two rounds of this (ten routes), while intermediate and advanced climbers can shoot for three or more rounds. You should be thoroughly exhausted when you're done.

TRAVERSE ELIMINATES

If you're new to endurance training, traversing is an excellent way to build a solid foundation. You can go as long or as short as you want, and because you don't get too high off the ground, you can step off the wall at any point. This is also an excellent active rest day exercise, as it will get you moving and using your muscles, but it's not too taxing on your body. Traversing is also very customizable. You can focus on one side of your body, certain holds, or specific fingers. Keep in mind that you will be using a large section of the climbing gym, so make sure you don't interfere with other climbers. It's best to do this when the gym is not too crowded.

The Workout

Use a near-vertical section of wall that will allow you to traverse for 20 to 30 feet—each traverse will be out and back, so you'll travel double the distance. Do this four times with a different eliminate each time—i.e., it will be "off-route" to use holds in

Game: Lucky Draw

Number of Players

1+

Setup

Write down ten different climbing moves onto slips of paper (drop-knee, right-hand lockoff, left-hand dyno, gaston, heel hook, etc.) and place the slips into a bag.

How to Play

Pull four slips out of the bag, and then try to create a problem or route that uses all of the movements.

Training Purpose

Sequence creation, creative thinking, unlocking beta, figuring out the benefit of one move versus another certain ways. First, traverse the section of wall using only sidepull handholds. All hand- and footholds are on, but you can only grip using the sides of the holds. The second traverse is a finger eliminate, meaning you use the same holds but only certain fingers on those holds; use only two fingers of each hand to grip (alternate the fingers if desired). Do the third lap using only the pinch grip on each hold. In the fourth and final set, traverse the wall using only one hand (e.g., use only the right hand out and only the left hand on the way back). This last round might require deadpointing or lunge moves to advance your hand from hold to hold. One-arm traverses take away the benefit of using the other hand to support you while you "feel out" a hold before weighting it, and force your muscles to engage quickly to keep you on the wall. This improves what is called reactive power, or your ability to increase holding power for specific finger and hand positions. When you encounter a tricky sloper or an awkward edge, you must make adjustments quickly. Rest three to five minutes between each traverse.

Game: Twister

Number of Players

Small groups of 3 or 4

Setup

This is similar to the popular board game. You can use the spinner board from the actual game or create your own selection system. Write on slips of paper: right hand, left hand, right foot, and left foot; and then the colors of holds (and types, for more of a challenge) on separate slips. One person is the "spinner." Climbers start on similar but separate sections of wall. It works best on vertical walls that are peppered with many holds, but it can be done on steeper terrain for a much harder challenge.

How to Play

The spinner randomly selects one of each slip. All climbers must then execute the movement (for example, left hand to blue crimp; right foot to green pinch). A player is eliminated when he cannot do the drawn movement.

Training Purpose

Flexibility, endurance, core stability

3X10 INTERVALS

If your inclination is to rest ("take" or sit back on the rope) when you're pumped, this workout is for you. It can be scary to climb when you're starting to feel tired, but if you don't push yourself past that threshold, you won't build more endurance. If you're a beginner lead climber, consider doing this on toprope until you get comfortable and skilled with taking lead falls. Doing it on toprope will eliminate the fear of falling and help you focus on training and trying hard.

The Four Types of Breathing

Breathing is a crucial component of climbing well, and there are four basic types. Think of them like gears on a manual car; they exist on a spectrum, from resting on a long sport climb to trying your absolute hardest for one bouldering move. The higher the gear, the more your core is engaged, but the faster you'll fatigue. Your breath is also a way of expressing intensity, which should match the difficulty.

Gear 1: Deep, Relaxing Breath

As it sounds, a deep breath when you're in a relaxed position on the wall helps you rest and reset your stress level.

Gear 2: Pffft!

Say it out loud. It forces air out of your mouth through pursed lips. This is the gear you'll be in for most moderate climbing. Breathing audibly helps remind you to keep breathing.

Gear 3: Ahhhh!

This is more of a scream. You are restricting airflow with your diaphragm to keep your core tight on a difficult move, but still breathing.

Gear 4: Hold Your Breath

To maximally engage your core muscles, you'll need to hold your breath fully. This should be done briefly and reserved for the hardest moves. Resume normal breathing as soon as possible.

The Workout

This format is three rounds of ten climbs in a row, and it's designed to help you tolerate the pump. Within each group of ten climbs, the highest difficulty should be one full number grade below your onsight level. The order should alternate easy–hard–easy–hard, with the hardest climbs in the second, fourth, sixth, and eighth slots; the tenth is a cooldown. The easy climbs should start about three number grades below your onsight, the next hard climb would be two number grades easier than your onsight. Choosing routes takes practice, so write down your groups beforehand so you don't have to keep track of them in your head. For a 5.11c onsight climber, it might look something like this:

(1) 5.8 (2) 5.9 (3) 5.8 (4) 5.10 (5) 5.9 (6) 5.10+ (7) 5.10- (8) 5.10+ (9) 5.9 (10) 5.8

Depending on how that felt, adjust the set to be easier or harder.
An easier group:
(1) 5.7 (2) 5.10 (3) 5.8 (4) 5.10+ (5) 5.6 (6) 5.10+ (7) 5.8 (8) 5.10 (9) 5.9 (10) 5.8

A harder group:
(1) 5.7 (2) 5.10- (3) 5.8 (4) 5.10+ (5) 5.7 (6) 5.10+ (7) 5.8 (8) 5.10+ (9) 5.9 (10) 5.6

Efficient Finger Training

Do weighted finger curls using dumbbells or a light barbell one to two times per week, along with the other strength-training exercises. Warm up with two sets using high reps / low weight, then perform three to five sets to fatigue using the reps listed below, then do two cool-down sets using high reps / low weight. Rest at least five minutes between sets. Stretch forearms thoroughly afterward.

Months 1 and 2: Twelve to thirty reps per set; light weight

Months 3 and 4: Three to eight reps per set; more weight

Months 5 and 6: Thirty seconds to one minute of continuous curls

Months 7 and 8: Twelve to thirty+ reps per set with light weight for maintenance

Month 9: Focus on sending your project and take a break from training finger strength.

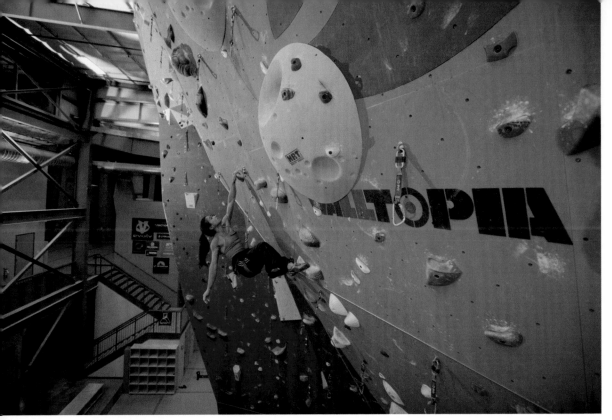

▶ *Up-Downs*

UP-DOWNS

Up-Downs, in which you climb up one route and down another, are a straightforward way to approach endurance training. But the downclimbing is no gimme—it should be a route that's moderately difficult for you. That way you work on technique simultaneously with endurance. It will force you to think about the strongest part of your body first: the feet and legs. Leading with your lower body is key to understanding movement and improving body awareness.

The Workout

Pick two adjacent climbs (boulder or sport) at grades you can flash, one slightly harder than the other. If you climb V7, pick a V5 and a V4. Climb up the harder problem first. Once you reach the top of the boulder, shake out, and without topping out or jumping off, downclimb to the start of the next problem using any holds on the wall. Without letting your feet touch the ground, complete the second climb and jump off or top out. Rest a few minutes and repeat for the rest of your climbing session.

GET STRONG FOR STEEP SPORT

While most people might jump right on the wall and crank out lap after lap at a comfortable grade, that type of training by itself won't really help you tick harder grades or improve on the steeper angles. Ten laps on a 5.10 will help build endurance at that grade, but when it comes time to work that 5.12 project, you'll be left wanting. The following is a simple, effective four-week training program that's designed to help you float the most wicked overhangs. The plan focuses on technique, endurance, core strength, power-endurance, and perhaps the most underestimated but important part of climbing overhangs—resting. If you've ever stared up at the steepest section of the wall in your gym and wanted to float up it like a pro, this program is for you. Do it four weeks any time you're looking for a program that will provide results but isn't too committing.

GUIDELINES

This four-week program is ideal if you've been climbing regularly and are in good shape. If not, start with four weeks of general climbing training to get back in shape. Aim to climb at least three times a week: bouldering, sport climbing, or a combination. Once you have this baseline fitness, begin the specific training outlined here.

▶ Shoot for climbing-specific training four days a week, in a two-days-on, one-day-off pattern. If you're feeling really tired, take more days off. Rest is just as important as training when you're going hard. Listen to your body.

▶ Because this is a shortened, discipline-specific plan, you should go hard in every session. You should work at 85 to 100 percent of your max every day.

▶ If you're already an endurance fiend, focus more on power-endurance and consider adding a campus board workout one day a week on an endurance-focused day.

▶ Each day has a climbing workout (power-endurance or endurance, followed by a specific focus for the day (technique, core, or resting). Pick one workout for both climbing and focus.

▶ Warm up every day with twenty minutes of easy climbing.

WEEKLY SCHEDULE

For the purpose of our example, we started our weekly schedule on Monday, but you can start on the day that works best for you, and then adjust accordingly. Repeat this weekly schedule four times, and dial up the intensity a bit for each consecutive week. Do this by incorporating harder bouldering problems and sport routes into your climbing days.

MONDAY
CLIMB: Power-endurance

FOCUS: Core

TUESDAY
CLIMB: Endurance

FOCUS: Technique

WEDNESDAY
CLIMB: Rest

FOCUS: Core

THURSDAY
CLIMB: Power-endurance

FOCUS: Resting

FRIDAY
CLIMB: Endurance

FOCUS: Technique

SATURDAY
CLIMB: Rest

FOCUS: Core

SUNDAY
CLIMB: Power-endurance

FOCUS: Resting

RESTING

1. Pick a steep route that's slightly easier than your redpoint max. Climb it once, and figure out where you can get at least two rests. This will help you identify what a good rest is and how to maximize it, as well as how to pace your climbing between rests. Now reclimb the route, and use those two rests for at least twenty seconds each. Arms should be straight, shoulders relaxed, and feet in the best position to take weight off your arms; heel hooks and the like are especially helpful. Focus on using minimal energy, getting your heart rate down, shaking out, alternating hands, and relaxing. Be mentally present when resting: How pumped are you? How does shaking out feel? If you move your foot slightly up or down, can you find a better position? Do this on two to three routes; if you fall off at any point, get back on and complete the route.

2. Create a twenty-move boulder problem loop on the steepest part of the bouldering wall. Have it start and end on the same big holds with good feet. Do the problem, and when you get back to the start, rest there without coming off the wall for a set amount of time; three minutes of resting is a good start. Focus on staying relaxed, breathing evenly, shaking out, keeping open hands, not over-gripping, etc. Try to complete the loop at least three times. The next week, create a new problem with a start end position that has good hands but slightly worse feet. The set resting time might feel too long, but this will get your brain in tune with your body and help you figure out not only how to use rests, but how long you should rest. Create two to three separate problems or loops for each session, aiming to complete each three times.

3. Choose an overhanging route at your absolute limit. Climb the route until you feel the pump creep in. Keep moving, and right before you feel like you're going to peel off, find a massive jug—even if it's not on your route—and milk that rest like there's no tomorrow. Get into the best resting position you can, using whatever holds are available. The idea is to push yourself to your physical limit and then get a break while not dropping off or coming down. Stay there as long as needed, and see how much strength you can get back. It's fine if you fall two moves later; that's two more moves than you would have done otherwise. This builds mental fortitude when resting, creates confidence, and helps you develop a positive attitude about resting. Try this with four routes, making sure to rest about ten minutes between each.

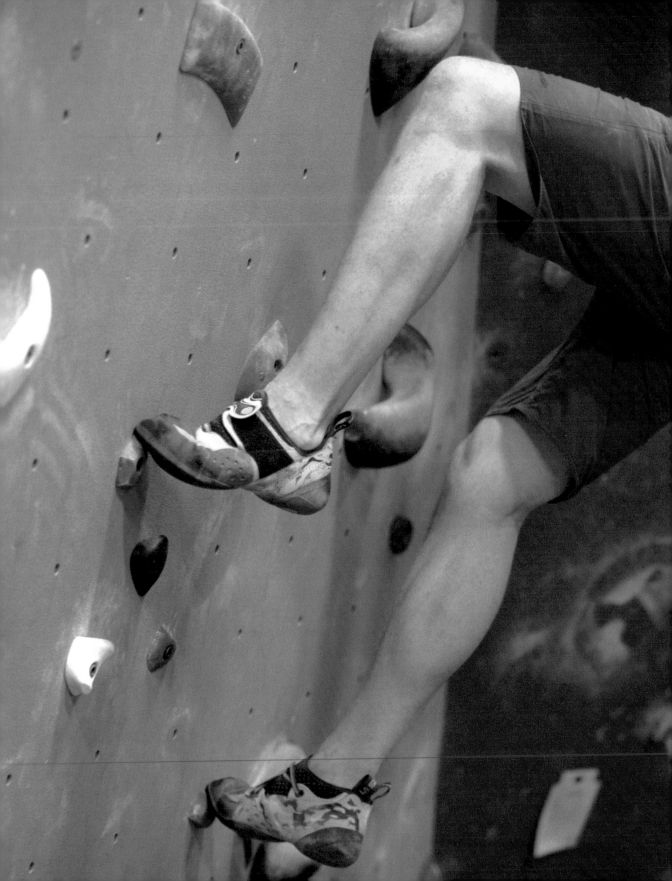

ENDURANCE

1. Laps are a great way to gain endurance quickly, but, with a limited number of routes in a typical gym, they can get boring really fast. Use this exercise sparingly so you don't burn out too quickly. Pick a route a full number grade below your max redpoint and climb it. Lower, pull the rope, and get back on the wall as fast as you can. You don't have to climb it fast, and you can (and should) rest on the route, but don't dillydally getting back on. Try to gain energy back while on the wall. Run three to five laps on a few climbs, doing a minimum total of twelve pitches.

2. Downclimbing is an underrated training exercise. Not only does it help with footwork and technique, but it also works your main climbing muscles in the opposite direction, like doing "negatives" in weightlifting, focusing on the lowering motion more than the upward motion. Pick a route that's a full number grade lower than your redpoint max and climb up. Immediately downclimb the whole thing, and without coming off the wall, start climbing back up. (An autobelay is great for this.) When you get to the top the second time, just lower to the ground. Do this on at least four routes.

3. Pick an overhanging route that's at least a full number grade below your redpoint max, the juggier, the better. Every time you want to reposition your feet, purposely cut both of them, swing them out, and bring them back to the wall in the position that's necessary to move upward. These are called Peter Pans (see page 43 for instructions). It should look something like this: Move right hand, move left hand, cut feet, swing them out, and as you bring your feet back to the wall, place them where they need to go to make the next set of hand movements. Do this on at least six routes, more if you're an advanced climber.

CORE

1. Do all exercises in a row, then repeat each set three to five times, with a 2-minute rest between each set.
   - 1-minute forearm plank
   - 30-second side plank (each side)
   - 1 minute of mountain climbers
   - 2-minute hip bridge
   - 10 leg raises on pull-up bar
2. Do all exercises in a row, then repeat each set three to five times, with a 2-minute rest between each set.
   - 1-minute bent-leg boat pose
   - 1 minute of bicycle crunches
   - 10 full sit-ups
   - 1 minute of flutter kicks
   - 20 airplanes (alternate sides)
3. Do all exercises in a row, then repeat each set three to five times, with a 2-minute rest between each set.
   - 1-minute straight-arm plank
   - 1 minute of Russian twists with medicine ball
   - 15 back extensions / Supermans
   - 1 minute of leg climbers (alternate sides)
   - 30 crunches

TECHNIQUE

1. Bouldering is one of the best ways to gain good technique quickly. Because the problems are short, you can focus on each move and the subtle nuances of footwork, body position, and how to grip slopey or small holds. You'll also simultaneously build power, which is often overlooked in sport climbing training but is just as necessary to be successful on challenging routes. Spend thirty minutes projecting hard boulders at your limit.

2. Work with a partner on the system board. Create problems (usually five to seven moves) that incorporate all different types of movement, holds, and body positions. Focus on your weaknesses, whether they're a certain type of hold or a

certain movement. Because a system board is mirrored, with the same holds in the same spots on each side, make sure to do every problem twice, once on each side. Spend thirty minutes creating problems for each other on the system board.

POWER-ENDURANCE

1. The classic workout to gain power-endurance is a 4x4. On a bouldering wall, find four problems about three grades below your redpoint max. Climb the first problem four times without resting, then rest two minutes and climb the second problem four times. Continue until you've completed one set. Rest at least five minutes and repeat the 4x4 with four new problems. Rest again and repeat with new problems for three total sets.

2. The Treadwall is one of the best climbing inventions since sticky rubber. Kick the angle back so that you can do four rounds in a row without coming off. Choose problems that are at least three grades below your max, and then time yourself doing four rounds (the same problem repeated or different problems, it doesn't matter). After the four rounds, rest 1.5 times the length of time it took you to complete the problems, so if it takes four minutes to do four rounds, rest six minutes. Do at least four sets of this. As you get stronger week by week, try to make the wall a little steeper.

3. Choose fifteen boulder problems about three grades below your max, and climb them all in thirty minutes or less—you should have to hustle. Rest fifteen minutes, and then climb them all again within thirty minutes.

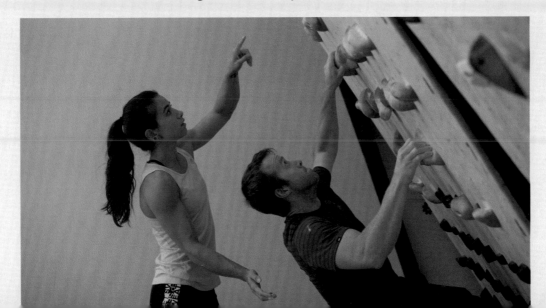

CLIMB 5.12

The 5.12 grade is considered an important benchmark for many climbers, and it's attainable for most 5.11 climbers who are willing to work for it. (If you're a 5.10 climber looking to jump to 5.11, you can follow the same guidelines—just knock the difficulty down on your climbs and training.) Whether it's strength or endurance or technique holding you back, the following plan provides guidelines to help you achieve your goal in nine months. Your mental game could also be holding you back, so make a concerted effort to master those areas (shaky confidence, fear of falling, lack of focus, etc.).

GUIDELINES

Climb

▶ Establish a weekly training schedule and stick to it.

▶ Climb two to four days/week, but never more than two days in a row.

▶ Warm up with light aerobic exercise, dynamic stretching, and easy climbing.

▶ Take at least one day of total rest each week.

▶ Focus on all types of holds, angles, and moves.

▶ Spend one or two first-days-on (your first day climbing after a rest) bouldering each week.

▶ Incorporate 4x4 power-endurance training one time per week. Climb four 12- to 20-move boulder problems four times each, with 1 to 5 minutes of rest between each problem.

▶ Incorporate high-intensity endurance training 1 to 2 times per week. Climb 3 to 7 routes with 20 to 25 pumpy moves to a resting hold. Shake out and recover, then climb for another 15 to 20 moves.

Strength

▶ Weight train two times per week right after climbing or the day after; don't climb to exhaustion and then weight train.

▶ Rest two days between each weight session.

▶ Day 1: Pull-ups / lat pull-downs; tricep push-downs / dips; rows; wrist curls; reverse wrist curls.

▶ Day 2: Deadlifts; squats; bench presses / push-ups; military presses; captain's chair leg lifts.

▶ Rest three minutes between sets of the same exercise.

▶ Do weighted finger curls one to two times per week. See the Efficient Finger Training sidebar (page 85).

▶ Do one set (lighter reps) of each exercise the last week of each month, and take extra rest days.

MONTH 1

CLIMB: This should be an even mix of bouldering and endurance days.

TECHNICAL FOCUS: Toprope or bolt-to-bolt several 5.12a routes. Select your project and begin daily route visualization.

STRENGTH: One warm-up set followed by two sets of eight to twelve reps to fatigue (meaning you can't do more than eight to twelve reps using the weight chosen). See Guidelines) for specific exercises.

MONTH 2

CLIMB: Same as Month 1.

TECHNICAL FOCUS: Quiet, precise footwork on small crimps and pockets. Watch your feet connect with every foothold.

STRENGTH: Increase weight as you gain strength.

MONTH 3

CLIMB: Same as Month 2.

TECHNICAL FOCUS: Keep your arms straight by bending your knees and lowering your hips. Practice this on small handholds and footholds; relax your grip.

STRENGTH: Increase weight so you reach fatigue at eight reps in sets two and three this month.

MONTH 4

CLIMB: High-intensity bouldering two times per week. Create boulder problems that mimic the crux movements on your project, but are a bit harder. Work problems one to two times per week. Decrease endurance days as needed for recovery.

TECHNICAL FOCUS: Lock off on small crimps and pockets on vertical or gently overhanging angles.

STRENGTH: One warm-up set, then one to six reps to fatigue for sets two and three.

MONTH 5

CLIMB: Same as Month 4.

TECHNICAL FOCUS: High step on small footholds on vertical/gently overhanging angles, plus lockoffs as in Month 4.

STRENGTH: Same as Month 4. Increase weight if possible.

MONTH 6

CLIMB: Decrease bouldering to one time per week and increase power-endurance and endurance. Include 4x4 training one time per week, and endurance training one to two times per week. Incorporate 5.12a crux boulder problems from the previous months into sport routes that mimic your project.

TECHNICAL FOCUS: Start breathing audibly on the ground, and breathe continuously while climbing. Return your breathing and heart rate to normal while shaking out at rests.

STRENGTH: Set the weight on pull-ups / pull-downs, triceps dips, and rows at a level where you can perform two sets of three to five reps quickly ("dynoing" the weight) while maintaining technique. Stop when you can't move the weight quickly. Maintain other lifts as in Month 5.

MONTH 7

CLIMB: Build up to repeating last month's project-simulation routes three to five times in a climbing session, one or two days per week. Continue bouldering one day per week; work power-endurance one day per week.

TECHNICAL FOCUS: Mentally rehearse the moves ahead while resting; move quickly and accurately through hard sequences, using precise footwork.

STRENGTH: Same as Month 6.

MONTH 8

CLIMB: Solidify your 5.11 base; aim to redpoint four 5.11c routes and three 5.11d routes that are similar to your project.

TECHNICAL FOCUS: On your first day on, do one to two burns on your 5.12a project. Note any areas that still need work. Visualize the moves daily.

STRENGTH: One to three sets of one to five reps for all lifts.

MONTH 9

CLIMB: Sending your project will likely take more than a day, and you can't put in more than two to three solid redpoint burns in a day. Have some secondary, easier projects to work on day two. If you want to try your project two days in a row, don't try anything hard after your attempts on the 5.12a. Instead, do a warm-down pitch, stretch, and call it a day. Let go of expectations and enjoy the process, learning everything you can from the route. Remember that climbing at your limit always includes more days of "failure."

TECHNICAL FOCUS: Establish a two- or three-pitch warm-up routine to help you judge whether you're recovered. The final warm-up should get your blood going, but not be so hard that you're pumped. Don't sabotage your day by going for the send first thing. Rest at least thirty minutes between redpoint attempts.

STRENGTH: Maintain a light training regimen so you don't lose your strength gains. Keep the volume low and the weights manageable; don't train to fatigue. If you're tired or sore from climbing, it's better to skip exercises and avoid injury.

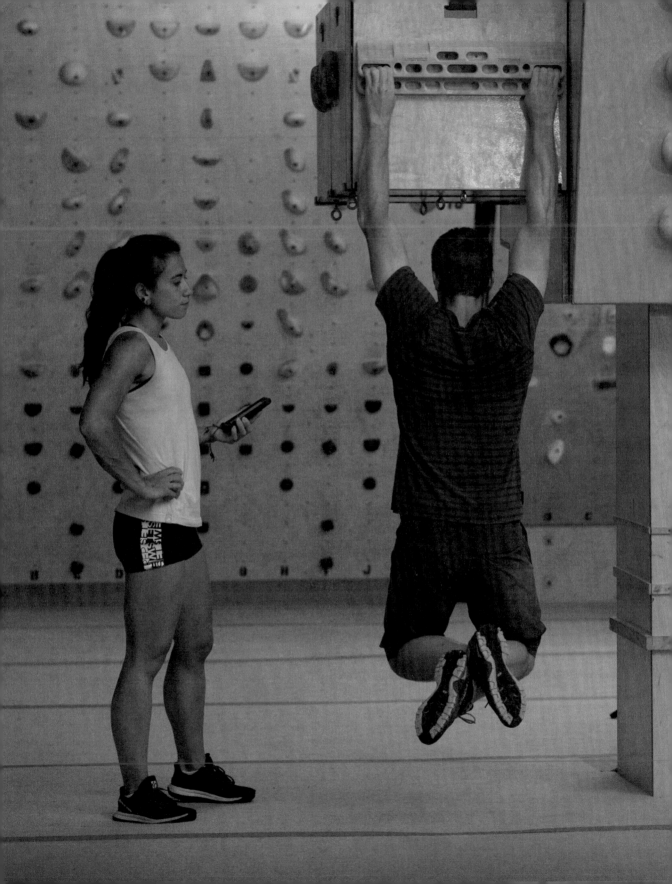

Chapter 4

CLIMBING SUPPLEMENTS

ESTABLISHING BASELINE CLIMBING FITNESS is best done by simply climbing, but once you get a good foundation, you might find you haven't seen any noticeable improvement in a while. This is called a plateau, and some climbers experience it within their first few months of climbing; others can climb for years and never reach a plateau. There are specialized tools in the training world designed to help you improve specific aspects of climbing strength: the hangboard, the campus board, and the system board. This chapter focuses on how to use each of these tools and other supplementary workouts, like pull-ups and injury-prevention exercises, to become a better climber.

You want to have a good foundation of strength in your arms, wrists, and hands before using these tools. Make sure you've done at least a few months of regular climbing before you try out these devices.

Similar to climbing holds, the hangboard, also called a fingerboard, is a molded piece of plastic or wood that has several different types of grips on it. The idea is to hang on certain holds for a set amount of time to build finger strength. Stronger fingers mean you can use smaller holds, and holds that felt unhangable before will feel more manageable. Technically, finger strength comes from the forearms, but it's important to have strong tendons and ligaments throughout your hands and wrists. Hangboarding will help develop these as well, but it's very important not to overdo it. If you feel any weakness or tweaks, stop hangboarding and consider climbing for a few more weeks to build overall strength.

The campus board is for intermediate to advanced climbers who have adequate finger strength. You shouldn't be campusing unless you've been climbing regularly for at least a year and have some experience with the hangboard. The campus board is a series of wooden rungs placed a set distance apart. The goal is to move between the rungs without using any feet. This improves power, or the explosive strength to make big moves when holds are far apart. It's particularly important for bouldering, but roped climbers find benefits from using the campus board too. Most gyms have rungs of different sizes and shapes, from big jugs to small edges, so you can choose what works best for you. Most gyms have edges below the campus rungs for your feet, so you can start with two feet on, then one, and eventually work your way up to true campusing.

The system board is usually a small, overhanging bouldering wall. It is an ideal way to train repeated technical moves because the layout of mirrored holds—meaning holds on each side of the board are identical—allows you to practice the same moves with both sides of your body. Usually the holds on a system board are poor or hard to hold, so you want decent finger strength before you use this tool. The system board is a great spot to work on technique, because you can make up specific moves that are hard for you and work them repeatedly.

All of the following hangboard, campus board, and system board workouts are specifically designed to help you climb harder, so keep that in mind if you're a beginner or are just interested in general fitness, these may be too specific. Most of these workouts take an hour or less, and the best time to do them is after a moderate climbing session. Make sure you don't climb to exhaustion, though; save some energy to make the most of this supplementary training. For example, you might want to do the Strength 4x4 (page 53) workout, and then do a hangboard workout, or the Endurance Laps exercise (page 81), and then a campus board workout. If you're short on time, feel free to do these workouts on their own, but you must warm your body and hands up with at least fifteen to twenty minutes of easy climbing first.

HANGBOARDING 101

If you're totally new to hangboard training, this is the workout for you. It will get you familiar with proper hanging position, and get those hands, wrists, and forearms strong for more challenging training in the future. The most basic exercise on the hangboard is the deadhang, meaning you simply hang from your selected holds. Good form on your deadhang will help you avoid injury. Hang with a slight bend in your elbows, and pull your shoulder blades down and back, keeping body tension high. Practice the form on jugs or a pull-up bar before using the board's smaller holds.

The Workout

Begin each session with a full-body warm-up. Jumping rope for five to ten minutes is an excellent option, or take a quick run around the neighborhood. Do a few pull-ups and a bit of shoulder and finger stretching to get the upper body ready. Use the board's jugs or a bar for the pull-ups; doing pull-ups from small holds puts you at risk for injury.

Game: Fast Fun

These games are less involved than others but are still interesting.

▶ **Compete with Your Belayer for Points**: V2 is 2 points, V3 is 3 points, etc. A fall costs you one point. Climb all night, and the highest number of points wins.

▶ **Pick-Up**: For the younger crowd, use stuffed animals or small coins. Prop them on holds and have the little ones climb until they've collected them all without coming off.

▶ **Forced Falls**: Climber and partner pick climbs they're pretty comfortable on. While one person is climbing, the partner yells "Fall" at any point, and the climber has to let go right then and there.

▶ **Tag**: A group spreads out on the wall and starts traversing. Each person tries to tag the person in front. If you get tagged, you're out; if you fall, go to the back of the pack and start over.

▶ **Single-Foot Sending**: Climb a problem with only your right foot, and then climb it with only your left.

Hangboard Adjustments

Three minutes of rest between sets is a suggestion. Take as much time as you need to feel completely rested and fresh. Resting longer won't compromise your workout; it will help you focus on targeting strength and not endurance. The quality of each hang is crucial. The goal is to be almost failing on the last rep of each set. This means the first hang will likely feel easy, and they'll get progressively harder until you think you'll fall. This can be difficult to find at your body weight on any specific hold, so you may have to experiment by adding or subtracting weight or choosing different holds. Use a pulley system to remove pounds; most gyms have them, so ask a staffer to show you how to use it.

Two or three thirty-minute workouts per week can deliver excellent results. Hangboarding puts a lot of stress on small muscles and tendons—that's the point—and this requires you to listen to your body as you progress through the workouts. If you can't finish a set, end the workout. If your fingers or elbows become sore, take a week off, reevaluate your deadhang form, and ease back into your next training session.

▶ Using an open-handed grip, grab a matched pair of holds with all four fingers. Hang for ten to fifteen seconds. If you can hang for more than fifteen seconds, use smaller holds; if less, use bigger holds.

▶ Rest one minute after each hang, and then hang again. Four hangs equals one set.

▶ Rest five minutes and do another set of hangs on the same holds or ones of similar challenge. Do four sets in all.

▶ After three weeks, increase the intensity by choosing holds you can only grip for five to eight seconds. This is the sweet spot for building strength; now that your body has adjusted to the stress of the hang, attempt to do every workout in this zone. (If you can't hold on for a minimum five-second count, use bigger holds.) As you become comfortable with the demanding nature of the smaller holds and shorter hang time, incorporate different holds into each set.

HANGBOARD REPEATERS

Fingers of steel are the foundation of harder climbing, so finger-strength training is an excellent addition to any climber's training regimen. Gains come from climbing with moves or holds that are taxing on the fingers, like bouldering at your limit, but the extraneous movement won't translate directly to finger strength. Max finger strength is your ability to grab a hold for five to ten seconds, and it is employed in lockoff cruxes or on moves that require latching tiny or slopey holds. Hangboarding targets this important element of climbing. Training strength usually requires isotonic exercises like pull-ups, which involve moving the joint through its range of motion so muscles get stronger at every angle. In climbing, the fingers remain relatively static after grabbing a hold, so it's best to train finger strength in the most common positions: full crimp (second knuckle above the first), half-crimp (second knuckle even with the first), and open hand (second knuckle below the first). To train those positions use isometric exercises, meaning holding a position statically without moving the joint (the deadhang).

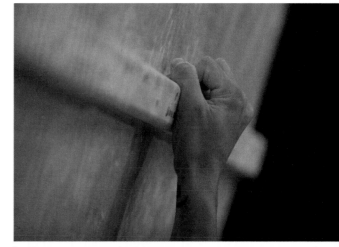

▶ *Finger position: Full crimp.*

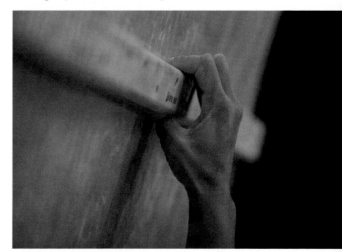

▶ *Finger position: Half crimp.*

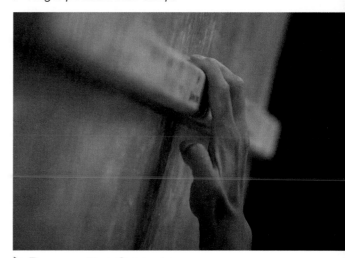

▶ *Finger position: Open crimp.*

You will gain strength in roughly 20 degrees of joint flexion in either direction from the grip you choose. Remember that hangboarding can cause finger injury if not performed carefully. Approach training conservatively.

The Workout

For a basic hangboard workout, do ten sets of five hangs on a variety of holds. To start, use a large edge, a small edge/crimp, a two-finger pocket, a three-finger pocket, and a sloper. Each hold will be used twice in a row, and every hold except the small edge will be done with an open-hand grip. Smaller holds can be used with the half-crimp or full-crimp positions, but the full crimp should be reserved for climbers experienced with training, as it's the most likely to cause injury. Even though hangboarding isn't as stressful on your fingers as campusing or hard bouldering, your muscles and joints still need plenty of time to recover. If it's your first time experimenting with hangboarding, try two workouts a week, making sure they're separated by forty-eight to seventy-two hours of rest. If this feels OK, move up to three workouts a week, but no more.

▶ Hold 1: 10-second hang, 5-second rest. Repeat the hang / rest cycle five times in a row, totaling 50 seconds on and 25 off, then rest 3 minutes.

▶ Hold 1 (same hold again, same grip style): 10-second hang, 5-second rest. Repeat the hang / rest cycle 5 times, then rest 3 minutes.

▶ Hold 2: 10-second hang, 5-second rest. Repeat the hang / rest cycle 5 times, then rest 3 minutes.

▶ Hold 2 (same hold again, same grip style): 10-second hang, 5-second rest. Repeat the hang / rest cycle 5 times, then rest 3 minutes.

▶ Continue with holds 3, 4, and 5, doing each twice for a total of 10 sets.

Progressing

After two to four workouts, you should find the last rep of each set to be a little easier, and you might not be failing on any of your last reps. This means it's time to up the difficulty. The best way to do this is by increasing the weight you're holding. It's easy to track, and doesn't require any additional testing for new holds. Add 1.5 to 2.5 pounds (lighter climbers try lighter weight; if that feels too easy, go for 2 or 2.5 pounds) to every set in your next workout. Do this by wearing a harness and strapping weight to the belay loop or tie-in points. Some folks use a weight vest, but that can actually change your hanging posture, which can lead to injury. You'll notice that early reps in a set will still feel about the same, but the last rep of each set will feel much harder. After another two to four sessions, the increased weight should feel easy again—that's when you'll add another 1.5 to 2.5 pounds. Continue with this system for four to six weeks. Most climbers will stop progressing somewhere around this point.

If you find it too difficult to add more weight after only three to four weeks, you've reaped the most efficient strength benefits you're going to get for now. Not everyone will progress the same, and it's best to cut your strength training once you have trouble improving. Consider moving on to another aspect of training, like power or power-endurance. If you want to keep building finger strength, take at least two weeks off from hangboarding before starting another four to six weeks of workouts. If that first cycle is all you want to do for now, don't worry. You won't lose much of your gains if you're bouldering or climbing at your limit at least once a week. You can add in some shorter workouts to make sure you keep that strength in the coming weeks and months. Pick three of the holds that gave you the most difficulty and continue doing one to two sets for each of those holds once a week.

CLIMB WITH GRACE ON THE SYSTEM BOARD

If delicate or balance-intensive moves are difficult, or you have trouble figuring out beta, consider fine-tuning your technique by targeting these moves on a system board. Practice is key. With enough repetitions, your brain stores those instructions in your muscle memory in little programs called motor engrams. These can work for or against you—if you ingrain bad habits, your climbing will reflect them. Learning and practicing the best ways to complete certain moves builds effective patterns that help you climb smoothly without thinking about it.

Your objective in training technique is to find new techniques to perfect and bad habits to fix. The more moves you practice and the more natural each one feels, the better you'll climb. This is especially important if your goal is to onsight and flash routes, where muscle memory is very important. Practicing with a partner is a great way to work technique, as she can spot flaws you don't notice. Ask your frequent partners if they've noticed any problems in your technique. Additionally, try filming yourself climbing to see what your weaknesses might be.

Technique can be trained during any session, but it should be done when you're fresh, on terrain that's easy for you. After you feel confident in your ability to do a move on easy terrain, try it on progressively harder holds. Eventually, you'll use those techniques on moves near your limit.

Game: Climb Like a Pro

Number of Players

1+

Setup

Pick a professional climber (or have a friend pick for you).

How to Play

Climb a route in the style of a specific pro climber. Use big dynos like Chris Sharma, static movements like Lynn Hill, or lots of technical trickery like Dave Graham. Choose athletes whose styles are different from your own.

Training Purpose

Working weaknesses, conscientious movement, experimenting with beta

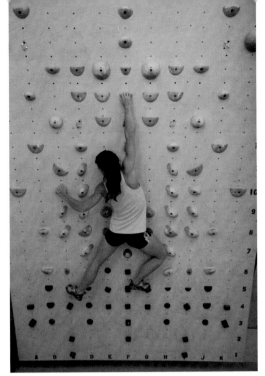

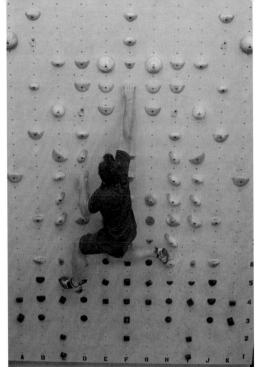

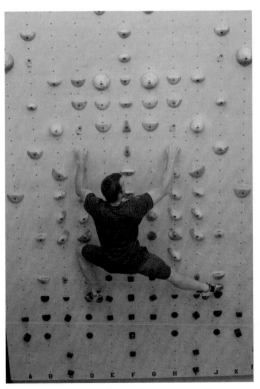

▶ *Practicing a variety of moves on the System Board.*

The Workout

To start, focus on lockoffs, drop-knees, and flags (see glossary for definitions of these movements). While you might be familiar with these moves, it's always possible to improve your technique at steeper angles or with worse holds, and each time you pull on, you'll gain a better understanding of the nuanced body positions required to do each move with the least amount of effort. Your first two sets will be lockoffs. Grab a large hold that's easy for you to hold with your right hand (beginner climbers will use larger holds, more advanced climbers will use smaller grips), and place the left foot on a small hold at waist height that's small enough to require at least some body tension. Pull on and reach as high as possible with your left hand, without touching a hold. Pay attention to how moving your hips and right leg affects how high you can reach, and how easy the move feels. Repeat this motion four times, resting in between if necessary. Take a few minutes of rest, then move to the other side of the board, which will work the other side of your body. Rest some more before following the same process with drop-knees and flags, pulling on and up to higher holds without touching them. After a session or two of this, start using smaller holds to make it harder. This is to "stress-proof" the techniques, meaning you can perform the moves under pressure. If you're working on a specific project, you can also dial in the crux moves by mimicking them on the system board.

MAKE BIG MOVES ON THE CAMPUS BOARD

Power equates to force over time—in movement terms, that means generating motion very quickly. When holds are far apart, getting from one to the next can require momentum, as well as the contact strength, to successfully latch once you've reached the hold. The campus board is the gold standard for training power. On vertical and slightly overhanging terrain, your legs, hips, and core generate most of the necessary power, but for steep boulders and routes, you'll need to rely on power from the upper body.

Increasing power requires several different muscular changes in your forearms, but they'll all be trained at the same time through the following approach. Broadly, the adaptations fit under the category of contact strength, which is how much force you can apply the moment you touch a hold. If you lack good contact strength, you might find it easy to slowly grasp a hold from the ground (using slow-twitch muscles), but can't grip the same hold during a dynamic movement, where you must latch it instantly (fast-twitch muscles). Training power forces your body to use more muscle fibers at once, as well as alters the types of fibers used from slow-twitch to fast-twitch.

The Workout

For a basic campus move, start with your hands matched on the lowest rail, exploding up to the next rail with one hand and grabbing it at the highest point of your movement. Jumping between rungs will feel uncontrolled at first, but keep your

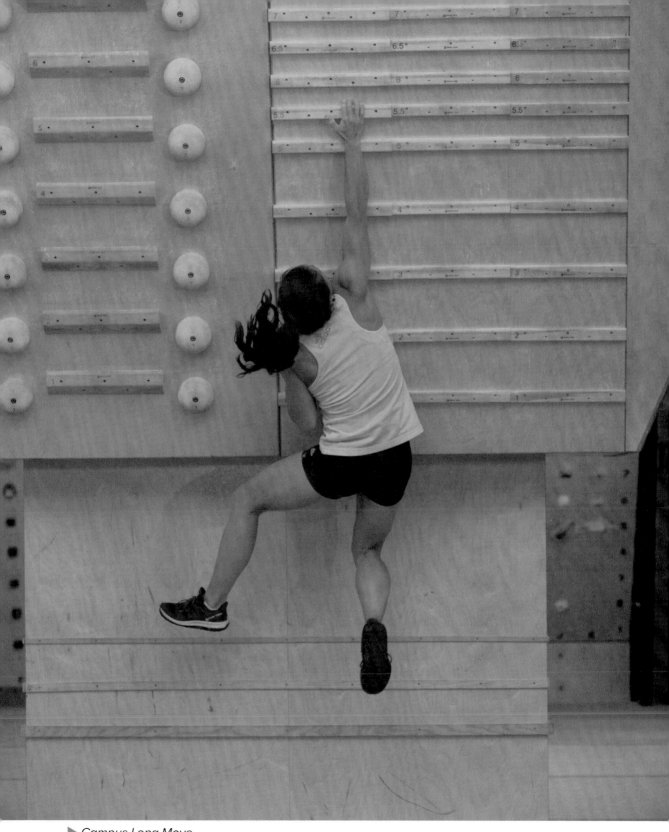

▶ *Campus Long Move*

Campusing Primer

To move between the spaced rungs, you must make explosive dynamic movements that are initiated by your upper body without the help of your feet, and then quickly latch the next rung. Starting out on the campus board, use the largest rails. You may need to use foot rungs to take some weight off your hands. The lower the foot rung, the easier the move will be. Eventually, the goal is to not use your feet. If you are using feet, focus on only resting your feet on the hold, not pushing with them. Pull with your arms, and keep in mind that you can change foot position throughout a session, moving to easier rungs as you get more tired.

core and legs tight, and maintain body tension throughout the move. Expect to latch the next rung, and you probably will. For your first workout, do four rounds of match ladders, followed by four sets of basic ladders. After each round rest two minutes, then switch the starting hand for the next round. Rest as much as you need to feel fresh for your next set.

After a few weeks, match and basic ladders may feel easy, so it'll be time to up the difficulty. Harder variations will train power in the arms and shoulders, while bumps will focus on contact strength. To start, do two sets of both matches and basic ladders, then two sets of harder ladders and bumps.

Keep in mind that training power can easily lead to injury, so workouts should be done when you're well rested and last no more than an hour, one to two times per week, with at least forty-eight to seventy-two hours of rest between workouts. Each exercise should only take ten to fifteen seconds, with rests between each activity. Longer rests will only increase your training's effectiveness and safety, so rest as much as you need to feel fresh. If any joint feels tweaky during a campus workout, or you feel you've lost your full power, end the workout.

▶ **Match ladders**: Start with both hands on the first rung. Move the right hand up one rung, then bring the left hand up to match it. Move the right hand up again, then match. (Switch the starting hand for each set.) Go as high as you can, then drop off.

▶ **Basic ladders**: Start matched on rung 1, move one hand to rung 2, then bring the trailing hand up to 3. Continue as high as you can, then drop off.

▶ **Harder ladders**: Start matched on rung 1 and move up to rung 3 with one hand, then rung 5 with the other hand. Repeat the move up to rungs 7 and 9 before dropping off.

▶ **Bumps**: Start matched on a rung around chest height. Bump one hand up one rung, and continue bumping it until you fail to latch the next rung. Do the same with the other hand. Pay special attention to your core and body position. Facing slightly left while bumping your right hand will feel more natural, and vice versa.

6-SECOND DEATH DROP

Don't be intimidated by the thought of training specifically for power; it's not as hard as you might think. If you're new to it and don't feel ready for the campus board, this is a great way to build a great base of power without risking injury. This short workout is perfect to tack onto the end of any gym session; it should take less than twenty minutes. The basic idea is to do pull-ups, but lower slowly. The lowering helps relieve stress off the tendons in the elbow; it stretches them after pulling all day. This type of eccentric training focuses on elongating the muscles, which trains the body to have greater control and focuses on building lockoff strength.

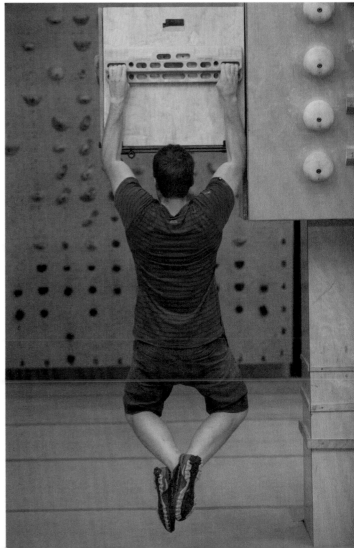

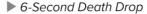 *6-Second Death Drop*

The Workout

- ▶ Find a pull-up bar, set of rings, or a hangboard.

- ▶ Do a pull-up and lower down slowly on a six-second count. You should not be at the starting position until the six seconds are up.

- ▶ Once you reach the bottom, pull back up as fast as you can and repeat the lowering process.

Sets: One to six pull-ups
Rest: Three minutes between each set
Reps: Five (or scale down to your ability)

PERFECT PULL-UPS

Perhaps no single training exercise elicits a more diverse range of opinions among climbers than the simple pull-up. Some swear by them, while others believe they are a waste of time. So what's the truth? Next time you're at the gym, watch somebody doing them. Typically, the motion starts with a jolt from the shoulders that throws the body upward. The instant momentum expires at the apex of the motion, the climber falls abruptly, bounces at the bottom, and repeats, until collapsing in a sweaty heap. This type of pull-up is fine if you're in a contest with your buddies, but it's nearly worthless for climbing training.

How to do an efficient and effective pull-up is broken down below, including several variations to target different muscle groups, so you maximize your training time and get stronger with one of the simplest exercises out there.

The Basics

Like most strength and weight training, the first rule for pull-ups is to forget quantity and focus on quality. The goal is to gain strength and control throughout the movement, which forces the smaller stabilizing muscles to do some work and get stronger. These smaller muscles are crucial for all climbers, whether you're dancing up a slab or trying to control a wild foot cut in the middle of a roof. When starting the motion, the first movement should be to engage the muscles by squeezing the shoulder blades together; don't just start from hanging on your skeleton. Between reps, return to this engaged position, not all the way down. Pull-ups train lockoff

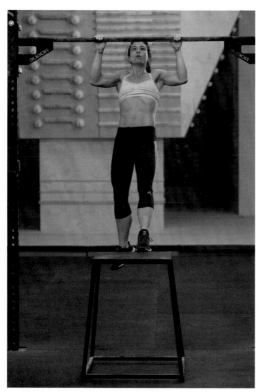

▶ Use a stool for assistance if you can't do a full pull-up yet.

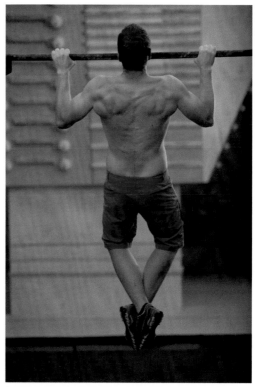

▶ The pull-up is a great upper body exercise for climbers.

strength and endurance for beginners and advanced climbers alike. Start with hands directly above the shoulders to work the lats, shoulders, back, and biceps. Working the hands wider forces a more difficult movement that engages the lats more. Shorter climbers will find these wide-grip exercises beneficial because they train for reachy moves and big lockoffs.

The Workout

Focus on climbing first, and then add pull-ups. Most people will get stronger just by climbing, so make that a priority and then add a few sets at the end of training days. Once you can do three to five sets of ten standard pull-ups, with three minutes rest between each set after a full session of climbing, consider rotating in sets of the pull-up variations listed below.

▶ **To get stronger on steeps**: Instead of your legs hanging straight down, elevate your lower body with boxes (or find a lower bar), so that with straight arms, your chest is facing the bar and your toes are pointing straight up with your body almost horizontal to the ground. Your heels should be on the boxes, or the ground if you are using a low bar. Pull your chest into the bar while keeping your body straight. Using the core to hold the body horizontal emulates an overhanging line, where the arms support most of the weight and create the power to move upward.

▶ **To get a more intense core workout**: Do pull-ups with your legs in a variety of positions. Try lifting your knees or, even harder, lift your straight legs so your hips are at a 90-degree angle. Too tough? Work separately to do L-hangs (hang from the bar with your legs extended horizontally), without a pull-up. Once you can do this for at least ten seconds, try it with a pull-up.

▶ **To get better at clipping**: Try Frenchies, which is an advanced technique that involves pausing at equal intervals in the motion. Pull up and hold your chin over the bar for a count of three (or five for more difficulty). Lower all the way down, pull all the way up, and then lower so arms are bent at 90 degrees; hold it for a count of three. Lower all the way down, pull all the way up, and then lower so your arms are two-thirds of the way straight (about 130 degrees); hold that for a count of three. Lower all the way down, pull all the way up, and then lower completely. That's one Frenchie. This develops the staying power to hold strenuous positions so you can figure out sequences or clip.

▶ **To get one-arm lockoff strength**: You can try a wide-grip pull-up, where your arms are much wider than shoulder-width apart. Another option is the towel (or uneven-grip) pull-up. Throw a towel, rope, or strap over the bar, putting one hand on the bar and the other about 18 inches lower on the strap. The initial movement should focus on pulling with the higher hand, but as you go up, you can start to push down with the lower hand. Less vertical distance between hands is easier; more is harder. Make sure to switch hands.

▶ **To get strong really fast**: Try weighted pull-ups, which you should only do if you can crank out ten quality pull-ups without coming off the bar. Start with five pounds for a few weeks, and work up as you get stronger. Anyone with shoulder injuries should be very cautious when doing weighted pull-ups, and it's probably best to avoid them altogether.

▶ **To gain endurance and strength**: Pull-up intervals will give you strength that lasts. The goal is to complete twenty one-minute pull-up intervals, each comprising a set number of pull-ups and a rest period taken within that one minute. Start with five pull-ups—you can do more or less depending on your strength level. Strive for a smooth, steady pace with perfect posture for each pull-up. After doing the five, dismount and rest for the remainder of the one-minute interval. At the start of the next minute, begin another set of five pull-ups. Upon completion, rest again for the remainder of the minute. Continue these intervals for ten to twenty minutes. If you make it to ten minutes, you will have completed fifty pull-ups in total—a great intermediate-level pull-up workout. If you make it the full twenty minutes, congratulate yourself for doing one hundred pull-ups. If you struggle to complete the ten minutes, then reduce the number of pull-ups per set to three or four. Conversely, increase the number of pull-ups to six or seven if the full twenty-minute routine feels anything less than grueling.

Game: Drag Race

Number of Players

Groups of 2

Setup

For boulder problems, set a timer for fifteen minutes.

How to Play

Go against the clock and your opponent by climbing as many problems as possible in the allotted time. Earn points for harder climbs: E.g., V3 is worth three points. Adjust accordingly to your gym's unique grading system (e.g., using spots). Whoever gets the most points wins.

Training Purpose

Endurance, power-endurance (and more fun than 4x4s!), climbing smoothly and quickly under pressure

Principles of Pull-Up Training

Dos

▶ **Move slowly.** Very few routes require cranking twenty-seven dynamic pull-ups in a row, but balance and static control initiated by the arms and back are crucial to nearly every climbing move. Slow down to the point where even doing ten pull-ups in one set is a challenge.

▶ **Go as high as you can.** The apex of the movement should put your chin well above your hands, which is a great way to train lockoff strength and get the most from your frame on long reaches.

▶ **Down is just as important as up—if not more so.** Aim for a one-second count on the upward portion, a brief pause at the high point, and then at least two to four seconds for the lower. The down portion is the eccentric phase, which contracts the muscles and simultaneously lengthens them—a more effective way to strengthen them.

▶ **Consider your equipment.** Standard workout bars are fine, but fingerboards and climbing holds are better. Jugs or big, flat holds are ideal; just remember you're working your pulling muscles, not finger strength.

Don'ts

▶ **Don't blast off.** A climbing move may begin from any point in the standard pull-up motion, and moves rarely start from a deadhang. That means every point of the motion is important to building climbing strength. Blasting off and relying on momentum negates its effectiveness.

▶ **Don't "kip."** A move popular among CrossFitters, kipping takes advantage of momentum to promote more reps.

▶ **Don't just drop your body weight onto straight arms.** Lower carefully back to the engaged-muscle position so you don't injure your shoulders.

▶ **Don't jump into it.** This minimizes the amount that the muscles you want to target (back, shoulders, arms, core) have to work, thereby reducing the effectiveness of the exercise.

▶ **Don't swing your legs or body.** Trying to keep from swinging becomes an exercise in itself, and will increase the movement's efficiency by upping how much you recruit your core.

FINGERBOARD MOVING HANGS

If your goal is to become a healthy, strong, and a well-rounded climber, then the ability to maintain composure through a difficult sequence on an endurance-based sport route is just as vital as the ability to muscle through a powerful move on a boulder problem. To help boost your endurance, supplement your gym training session with this simple hangboard workout once a week.

The Workout

Moving hangs involve working your hands around a fingerboard to produce a pump while working your finger strength. Using all holds on the fingerboard, create and follow a pattern for several minutes, moving one hand at a time. Include holds that exploit your weaknesses, like slopers or pinches. Don't deadhang; instead, your feet should support you while you're moving your hands. Mount a few foot jibs or wooden beams below the fingerboard, or position a chair or stool several feet behind the board, depending on your setup. Begin on comfortable starting

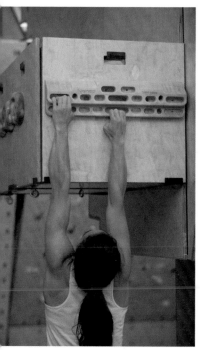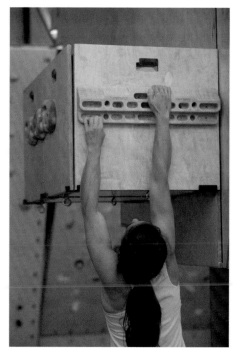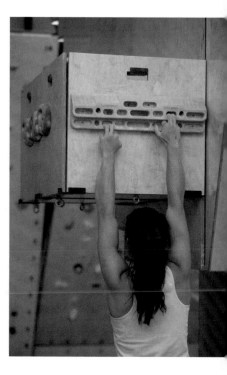

▶ *Moving between holds on a fingerboard.*

If You Can't Do a Single Pull-Up . . .

The best way to get better at pull-ups is to . . . do pull-ups. If you can't manage to crank off even a single rep, there are a few cheats that allow you to strengthen those muscles and eventually do them without help. You can also incorporate these methods to finish full sets of ten when you're tired.

▶ Have a friend help push you up and take some of the weight, just like getting a "power spot" when climbing. Have your helper stand behind you and put her hands on your hips. As you pull, she should try to lift you up, assisting you through the motion.

▶ Use a chair. Place it in front of you so you can reach it with one foot through the entirety of the pull-up motion. Do the exercise with one foot pushing off the chair; as you get stronger, you can move the chair farther and farther away, which means there's less weight on the chair and more on your arms. Eventually you won't need the chair at all.

▶ Try the pull-up machine, which simulates the movement while you stand on a platform that moves up and down to provide counterweight. As you get stronger, use less weight. If your gym doesn't have a pull-up machine, try doing lat pull-downs, which develop the necessary pulling muscles.

▶ Loop a TheraBand (a stretchy, wide rubber band used for adding resistance to movements, or in this case taking some of the weight) over the pull-up bar and tie a loop in it you can slip your feet into. Pull with your arms and straighten your leg to "stand" in the loop, so it gives you a small amount of support. These stretchy bands have varying degrees of resistance, so use a higher-resistance band for more assistance.

holds—usually the largest jugs—and move your hands around the fingerboard, holding each hand position for three to five seconds. Your goal is to stay on for at least five to ten minutes. Once you begin to feel the pump, move back to the large holds and shake out each arm for about thirty seconds. When rested, begin moving around the board again. When you've reached your time goal, rest for five to ten minutes before proceeding with a second and third set. Aim for three sets per workout, twice a week.

LADDERS ON THE BACHAR LADDER

Our fingers do a lot of work while we're climbing, and many climbers are obsessed with finger-strength training. But all the finger strength in the world isn't going to translate to harder sends if you haven't worked on developing the power to crank your body weight up off those tiny holds your iron tendons might be capable of crimping. John Bachar, a groundbreaking climber who made a name for himself in the 1970s and '80s, was forward-thinking in his training techniques, and developed the Bachar Ladder to develop stronger upper body and lockoff strength. A Bachar Ladder comprises evenly spaced dowels (or PVC pipes covered in grip tape) tied to a rope hung on a diagonal angle. By ascending the dangling ladder without the use of your feet, the instability of the tool forces you to use your core, shoulders, and back for stability.

The Workout

Not all gyms have Bachar Ladders, but if yours does, take advantage of it. Consider doing this to train power if you have had past finger injuries. Do this workout after

Prevent Finger Injury

Only climbers with healthy fingers should hangboard. Newer climbers and those with past finger injuries should pay close attention to how each digit and joint feels during each session, and back off if anything feels suspect.

To warm up before hangboarding, do at least twenty minutes of easy bouldering or route climbing, making sure to slightly ramp up the intensity so your fingers work harder gradually. If you can't climb to warm up, you'll have to improvise. Any grip-strength trainer—a malleable stress ball or putty, for example—is a good way to start warming up your fingers, but it's not a bad idea to do a short jog or some push-ups and core exercises to get the blood flowing. Before starting your workout, do some ten- to fifteen-second hangs and pull-ups on the largest holds on your hangboard to warm up your fingers. Do several easy, long hangs before beginning short hangs on slightly harder holds. Aim to play around on your hangboard like this for ten to fifteen minutes.

a climbing session; once a week is ideal. For safety, it's ideal to have a partner to spot you. Monitor your elbows and shoulders for pain during training—or if you feel labored gripping items, shaking hands, or lifting things with your shoulders. Tendonitis and soft-tissue strains and tears are not uncommon with this type of intense training. Gaining power will serve no purpose if you're injured.

▶ From the bottom of your Bachar Ladder, campus up one rung, match, and then campus back down to the bottom rung and match there.

▶ Step off and rest.

▶ Without matching on the second rung, campus to the third, match, and then down-campus back to your starting position.

▶ Step off and rest.

▶ Repeat incrementally by adding one rung with each set until you get to the top, then go back down, subtracting one rung at a time, like a pyramid.

TARGETED OPPOSITION

Tendonitis. Like it or not, if you're an avid climber, at some point you'll feel that deep, dull ache in your elbows or shoulders, a sign of inflamed tendons. The constant tugging is what does us in: using loads of pulling muscles (lats, shoulders, biceps, forearms) while neglecting the pushing muscles (pectorals, anterior deltoids, triceps), thus placing unidirectional strain on your tendons. If you mostly climb steep stuff, you're especially susceptible. As with all things in life, the key is balance. With these few simple stretches and weight routines, you'll balance the pushing and pulling muscles and increase mobility, thus enhancing your abilities and preventing injury.

The Workout

These exercises are really simple and require minimal equipment, so you can do them at home. Aim for two to three times a week on rest days.

▶ **Forearm Pronation/Supination**: Overusing the forearm's finger flexors and pronators often causes elbow pain (epicondylitis). The following exercise builds strength, as well as range of motion (i.e., let the weight stretch your forearms). Hold one end of a three- to eight-pound dumbbell vertically, with your elbow

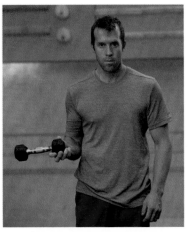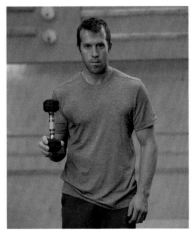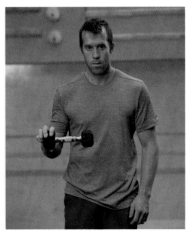

▶ *Forearm Pronation/Supination*

bent at 90 degrees and your upper arm by your side. Let your forearm rotate clockwise so that the weight drops outward and your palm faces the ceiling; hold for five seconds. Now reverse the rotation so your palm faces the ground; hold for five seconds. Complete two sets of fifteen reps, cultivating a comfortable fatigue by the final few repetitions.

▶ **Finger / Wrist Flexor Stretch**: Place your palms flat on the ground, a tabletop, or even against a wall, fingers facing toward you. Lean back to flex your wrists until you feel a comfortable stretch. Hold thirty seconds or longer, repeating two to three times.

▶ **Pec Fly with Shoulders on Physioball**: This exercise strengthens pectoral (chest) muscles, as well as the core and stabilizing muscles in your shoulders. Assume a bridge position, head and shoulders relaxed on the ball. Begin with a midweight dumbbell (10 to 20 pounds), arms fairly straight, palms facing each other. Slowly drop your hands ground-ward until they stop at or below shoulder height. Smoothly return them to their starting position; aim for three sets of twelve reps.

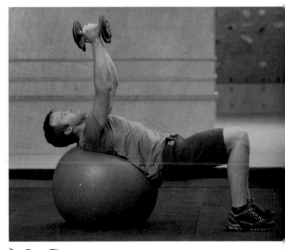

▶ *Pec Fly*

▶ **Latissimus Dorsi Stretch**: Lats, the primary climbing muscle in your back, can get really tight, creating hunched shoulders and back pain. To loosen them, stand in a doorway and hook the fingers of your right hand on the frame; now step back 2 to 3 feet with your right foot and bend forward. Look under your right armpit until you feel a comfortable stretch. Hold thirty seconds or longer, doing two to three stretches on each side.

▶ **Reverse Butterfly:** To support the often-overtaxed shoulder joint, you need strong rotator-cuff muscles. This exercise will get you there, while also promoting good posture, which is crucial to shoulder health. The prime muscles worked here are those in the backs of your shoulders: the rear deltoids, external rotators, and

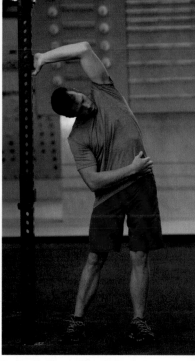

▶ *Latissimus Dorsi Stretch*

rhomboids. Begin with light dumbbells (5 to 10 pounds), hands together in front of your hips, elbows slightly bent. Draw your "butterfly wing" by bringing your hands up and diagonally outward, to finish with your elbows at shoulder height, hands facing forward. Now set your shoulders back and down, and bring your hands back to rotate your arms externally and complete the motion. Finally, with good control, reverse the motion by bringing your hands forward, down, and in, back to their starting position. Keep your torso stable and your shoulders pulled away from your ears at all times. Aim for three sets of fifteen reps.

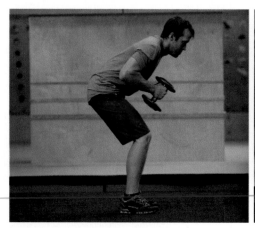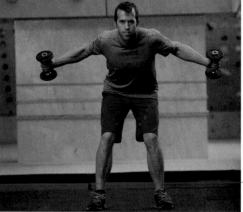

▶ *Reverse Butterfly*

SHOULDER ROUTINE

Shoulders are one of the most common problem areas for climbers. While climbing employs the larger muscles in the shoulder, the smaller stabilizing parts of the rotator cuff are ignored. Climbers must take the time to train these muscles so they're solid and reliable when it comes time to use them. These three exercises—the internal, external, and elevated rotations—are designed to keep your shoulders strong and happy. Try to do this super-short routine a few times a week.

The Workout

Do fifteen reps for two to three sets each, with no rest between exercises but a one-minute rest between sets. Start with an easy band and slowly work up. You're aiming for a nice even burn in your shoulders after the last set. If your band is too heavy, you're targeting the wrong muscles.

▶ **Internal rotation**: With the elbow tucked into your trunk, pull the band across your body. Transition right into external rotation.

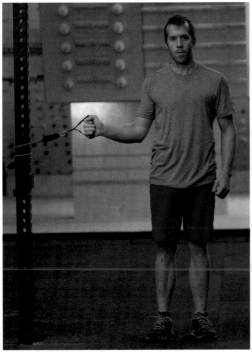 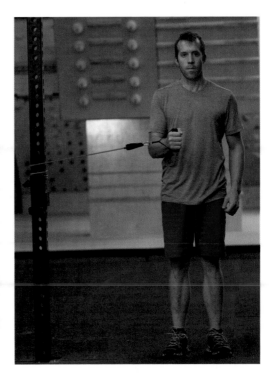

▶ *Band Internal Rotation*

▶ **External rotation**: Keep your elbow in the same place and pull the band out away from your body.

▶ **Elevated rotations**: You may use a band for these, or not. With elbows straight out and bent at 90 degrees, your palms should face the floor. Rotate at your shoulders to lift your hands so your palms face forward, then lower again to face the floor.

WRIST ROUTINE

When hangboarding, the wrist is a weak point. The forearms are bulky with muscle tissue, but the tiny ligaments and tendons of the wrist need to get special attention. These four exercises—the wrist rotation, curl, extension, and roller—are designed to keep your wrists strong and happy. These will take ten minutes or less, so do these at least once a week after climbing (twice is better).

The Workout

Do two to four sets of fifteen reps each. Pick a weight (start with 5 pounds) that will give you an even burn after the last set.

▶ **Wrist rotation**: Support your arm on a bench, and spin the dumbbell side to side.

▶ **Wrist curl**: Drop the weight all the way down and spin it back up.

▶ **Wrist extension**: You might need a lower weight for this. Lift the back side of your wrist up and drop it back down in a controlled fashion.

▶ **Wrist roller**: A wrist roller is a PVC pipe with a string through it and a weight on the end. Hold it straight in front of you with elbows slightly bent. Spin the weight up so the string wraps around the PVC pipe. Hold it there for a beat and then reverse it back down. Repeat that up-down motion once more.

PROTECT YOUR ELBOWS AND SHOULDERS

The repetitive motions of climbing and training are hard on the body. The sport involves lots of pulling down and pulling in toward the body, and the required muscles become well developed at the expense of other muscle groups. Add in common daily activities, such as sitting hunched over a desk or driving, and the potential for problems gets even worse. The result? Extreme wear and tear on the elbow and shoulder joints. But you don't have to be doomed to a future of physical therapy. By doing this small circuit of exercises, you can help prevent and even heal elbow and shoulder injuries.

The Workout

Do these daily or whenever you have a free moment—you don't have to sacrifice a chunk of climbing time. None of these exercises requires any equipment, so you can do them while working at your computer or watching TV.

▶ **Eccentric wrist curls**: Eccentric contraction means that the muscle-tendon unit lengthens under tension (similar to how your leg muscles lengthen under

Hangboard Ladders: A Few Rules

▶ Don't get pumped. If you are pumped or sweaty, you aren't resting long enough between hangs.

▶ Don't be in a hurry to get strong fast. Quick strength gains lead to quick losses. Slow gains are the ones you keep. Research shows that high-intensity training can lead to quick strength increases, with the gains coming from improvements in energy system efficiency. However, a slow, steady progression creates more efficient neurological pathways, which leads to persistent long-term gains.

▶ Only increase the load once a month. Don't look at strength training as an event or something to do this month, but as a new lifestyle habit. Your mind should not be on next weekend, but on five years from now.

▶ This training program can be used year-round. However, many climbers find that training constantly is difficult. For such climbers, try two four-week cycles, followed by a month of just climbing. After this "month off," resume the cycle. A good schedule is to train Monday and Thursday or Tuesday and Thursday. The specific days of the week don't matter, but you should have at least one day between training finger strength so you're fresh.

tension when you squat). It is key for this exercise not to load the tendon during the concentric phase (the muscle-shortening or curl part of the exercise). You can use a dumbbell if you like, but it's more convenient to press on a surface like a table edge. Resistance in this exercise should be heavy enough to provoke mild pain in existing injuries; gentle pain or discomfort is the goal. Bad existing injuries only need light pressure; mild cases may need to press fairly hard. If pain levels increase throughout the workout, dial it back. You're going too hard. For existing injuries, doing large numbers of reps (180 to 250 every day) gives better results than doing fewer reps. Fortunately, it's not much of an effort to clock up this sort of volume, because you can do the workout while sitting at a desk. It's also a good idea to do these exercises as prevention, especially if you have experienced an injury in the past.

1. With a straight arm, place three straightened fingers on the edge of the desk with your wrist pointing down (so the wrist flexor is shortened). Press into the table and, while maintaining firm pressure, allow your wrist to drop slowly, lengthening the wrist flexor through its whole range of motion. As your wrist extends, you should be able to provoke some pain in the tendon near your inner elbow (medial epicondyle) if you have a pre-existing injury.

2. Once you reach the end position with your wrist fully extended upward, bring your wrist back up to the start position—*under no load, without pressing into the table*—and repeat in sets of fifteen. Reduce the force you apply if the pain gets significantly worse as you work through sets. Eccentric contractions of this intensity are not really tiring, so you need very little rest between sets— have a sip of coffee and do another set.

▶ **Tennis Elbow Wrist Curls**: This exercise is the exact reverse of eccentric curls, and it is more easily performed with a dumbbell, heavy object, or by providing resistance with your other hand. Again, only apply the load during the eccentric phase, so if you use a dumbbell, use your other hand to pull it back up.

1. With straight arms, turn your wrist down, rest it on your knee, and place the other hand on top.

2. Pull your wrist upward into extension by moving the back of your hand up and toward you while adding pressure with your other hand to load the extensor tendon. If you're using a weight, simply grip it in your hand and do the same motion. If you have tennis elbow, you'll feel pain near the lateral epicondyle on the outer elbow. Again, many reps and a little mild pain are the order of the day. Remember to reduce the intensity if the pain increases through the workout.

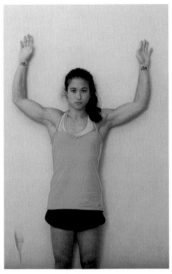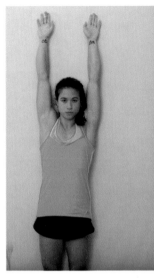

▶ *Wall Slides*

▶ **Wall slides**: This basic exercise to correct shoulder alignment and movement looks too easy until hunched, muscular boulderers try to do it. It stretches the internal rotators and promotes good activation and alignment of the entire shoulders.

1. Stand with your back resting against a wall, feet 3 inches from the wall and shoulder-width apart. Extend your arms upward, over your head. With elbows locked and arms pointing vertically, try to hold your arms against the wall. Most women will wonder what the problem is, while male boulderers will suddenly realize how limited their movement is due to their shortened lats. Hold your arms overhead for ten seconds, trying to push them as close as you can to the wall. This will feel very strenuous if your alignment is poor.

2. Now, keeping your forearms as close to the wall as possible, bend your elbows to 90 degrees, rotating your upper arms to horizontal. Your forearms should still point vertically. As you draw your arms down to this position, it will be difficult to keep the forearms from rotating outward from the wall if you have weak and poorly aligned shoulders. Do as many reps as you can; at least three per day as part of your warm-up is a good base.

HANGBOARD LADDERS

In climbing, when your fingers fail, the rest of your body fails. Focusing on this direct connection to the wall can benefit your climbing performance greatly, and luckily finger strength is relatively easy to train. The key is to do these correctly and in the right amount, as too many can be time-consuming, boring, and possibly harmful. This four-week program is great to do any time you're just climbing for fun, or doing the single workouts we provide in the Strength and Endurance chapters. Since it's not high-intensity, you can do it at the end of a climbing day. Hangboard ladders build long-term finger strength while staying far from the zone where injury is possible. The idea is to strategically change the volume of work in any given session, where easy, medium, and hard sets are cycled through and weights are adjusted in a way that increases strength while completely avoiding risk.

BEGIN HERE: FINGER POSITIONS

One school of thought for hangboard training is that you should always train an open-hand grip, but that doesn't mimic real-world climbing. Instead, this program focuses on three positions: open hand, half-crimp, and full crimp. They are the most common used in actual climbing, and they address the principle of "joint angle specificity." This principle says that isometric strength is gained only in a small range outside the angle in which it was trained. By covering all three positions, you are guaranteed to gain strength in any hand position you might encounter on the wall. No matter how disciplined you are about trying to hold an open-hand or half-crimp position (see page 103), when the going gets tough, the full crimp comes into play. The idea is to train this position carefully in a controlled environment instead of rolling the dice when on the wall.

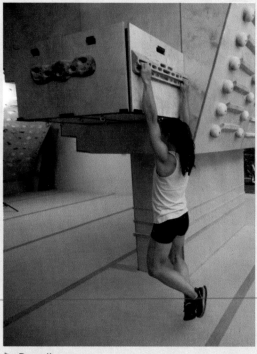
▶ Deadhangs

Open hand: Second joint is below the level of the first joint on a large edge or sloper; requires the least amount of effort

Half-crimp: Second and first joints are even on a hold; requires moderate effort

Full crimp: Second joint is above the first joint, requires the most effort

	1. Open Hand	2. Full Crimp	3. Half-Crimp
Week 1 (2 times)	3 sets of 3-6-9	3 sets of 3-6-9	3 sets of 3-6-9
Week 2 (2 times)	4 sets of 3-6-9	4 sets of 3-6-9	4 sets of 3-6-9
Week 3 (2 times)	5 sets of 3-6-9	5 sets of 3-6-9	5 sets of 3-6-9
Week 4 (2 times)	3 sets of 3-6-9-12	3 sets of 3-6-9-12	3 sets of 3-6-9-12

The Workout

1 **FIND AN OPEN-HAND GRIP** that you can hang onto for ten to twelve seconds. You can add or reduce weight, but it's best to start with a hold that you can hang on at body weight. For the next four weeks, this will be your training hold, so choose the hold carefully. Using this position, hang for just three seconds.

2 **REST A WHILE;** somewhere between ten and sixty seconds is fine. The actual time isn't important. The rule of thumb in strength is this: Long rests lead to great gains in neurological factors such as recruitment and firing rate; shorter rests lean more toward hypertrophy (muscle growth). Stay fresh to get strong. To fight boredom and continue resting, stretch, or complete another non-finger exercise.

3 **FOLLOW THE REST WITH** a six-second open-hand hang. Rest again, longer if you need to. Follow this rest with another hang, this time nine seconds long. After the nine-second hang, you've completed one ladder of 3-6-9. The beginning of the program starts with three sets of 3-6-9 ladders for each hold position. Rest as needed between sets. Repeat this pattern with a full crimp, and then finish with the half-crimp, also for three sets of 3-6-9. The full crimp is trained second to ensure you're warmed up for it. Finish with the half-crimp because it is the strongest position. Execute these moves well, remembering quality over quantity.

4   **DO THIS SESSION ONCE MORE** during the week. In the second week, increase to four sets per hand position twice a week. In the third week, do five sets per hand position twice a week. In the fourth week, do three sets for each position, but add a twelve-second hang so you are doing 3-6-9-12 twice a week.

5   **AFTER COMPLETING THE FOURTH WEEK,** assess your strength, and then restart the program with slightly increased loads, meaning add some weight to your hangs. Big load jumps aren't necessary, so add weight conservatively. If you add somewhere around 2 to 5 percent of your body weight each cycle for several cycles, that's great. The ultimate goal is to continue to progress over the long-term, and adding too much weight too soon will only result in a plateau.

How Isometric Training Works

The most basic way to get stronger is to work against a load that is "maximal" for just one or two repetitions. Training close to your max yields the greatest gains in strength, but there is a major problem: The body can't take it. Working with maximal loads takes a massive toll on the muscles and nervous system, and it also risks injury to joints and tendons with intense repetition. Moreover, recovering from training with heavy weights can take seventy-two or more hours, whereas training with a more moderate weight only requires about twenty-four hours to recover.

This is particularly true in isometric (static) training, where the exercise involves holding a muscle in a static position, like planks, wall sits, or hangboarding. Isometric training simply teaches the muscle to get strong in a fixed range; the muscle is not significantly lengthening or shortening during the set of work. This is in contrast to more "traditional" modes of training, called isotonic training, that involve concentric and eccentric contractions. Closing the elbow and bringing the weight up in a bicep curl, which shortens the muscle body, is a concentric action. The eccentric action—in this case, opening the elbow in a biceps curl—is the opposite, where the muscle is allowed to lengthen under load, as in opening the elbow in a bicep curl. Isometric action would simply be holding the elbow in one position, say a 90-degree bend. Although all three actions are used in most movement, climbers generally keep the fingers in a fixed position once they grab a hold, making isometric training the most useful for finger strengthening.

DIGIT DIALING

When it comes to tenuous pocket holds, it's especially important to prep the muscles and tendons that run through your fingers, hands, and forearms. This twelve-week program, designed for beginner and intermediate climbers, will give you stronger hands and fingers by increasing the intensity gradually. This is an intense finger workout, so only do this on days where you're fully warmed up from easy climbing but not that tired. While you can do another easy or moderate workout for the day, this workout is the main event, so save your energy and strength for it. This program is unique because instead of hanging with four fingers all the time, you'll hang with certain "teams," or pairs of fingers, at the same time (e.g., the pointer and middle finger). By using teams, you'll emphasize training the selected fingers instead of the whole hand. Advanced climbers can adapt it by using only one finger per exercise, rather than using finger teams. Teams are as follows:

Team 1: index/middle
Team 2: ring/middle
Team 3: ring/pinky

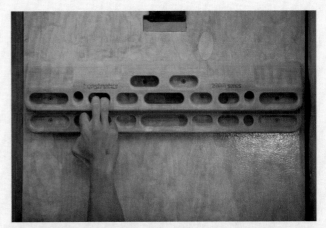

▶ *Finger Team 1*

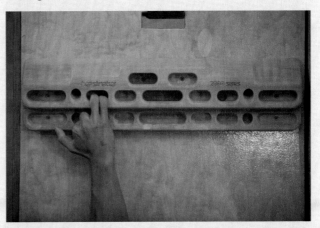

▶ *Finger Team 2*

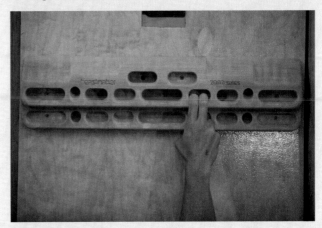

▶ *Finger Team3*

1. Finger Board/Campus Board/Systems Board

You can choose one or all three systems for this dead-hang exercise. When hanging, keep a slight bend in your elbows, pull your shoulder blades down and back, and use an openhanded grip—no crimping. Body tension should be high.

2. Dynamic Webbing Curl

Girth-hitch a piece of webbing around the necessary weight. Cycling through finger teams, slowly bend your fingers to "pick up" the weights, similar to how a bicep curl works. See chart for reps.

3. Levering

This exercise increases wrist and finger strength together. Begin with your forearm resting on your knee and your hand wrapped around the base of a lever (small sledgehammers work great, but anything with extra weight on one end works). The closer your hand to the base, the harder the workout. Rotate your wrist 180 degrees, left to right, for the number of reps specified in the chart.

***Terms from chart:

R/r: Uppercase "R" indicates resting for the remaining minute. Lowercase "r" indicates resting for 10 seconds after each exercise.

1 Pad/2 Pads: Use your judgment when deciding how deep a training hold or campus rung to use. One pad will provide a harder workout, while two pads is easier and safer for those just starting out.

Percentage of RM: This indicates a percentage of the heaviest weight with which you can do one repetition. For example, if your maximum weight for 1 rep is 20 pounds, and the chart calls for doing 8-12 pulls with 55 percent of RM, do 8-12 reps with 11 pounds.

The Workout

Apparatus	Finger/Team	Pocket Depth	Month 1				Month 2				Month 3			
			Week 1	Week 2	Week 3	Week 4	Week 1	Week 2	Week 3	Week 4	Week 1	Week 2	Week 3	Week 4
1 Finger Board Campus Board Systems Board	Team 1	1 Pad/2 Pads	20s	23s	27s	30s	7s R	8s R	9s R	10s R	7s r	8s r	9s r	10s r
	Team 2	1 Pad/2 Pads	20s	23s	27s	30s	7s R	8s R	9s R	10s R	7s r	8s r	9s r	10s r
	Team 3	1 Pad/2 Pads	20s	23s	27s	30s	7s R	8s R	9s R	10s R	7s r	8s r	9s r	10s r
	1 Finger	1 Pad/2 Pads	20s	23s	27s	30s	7s R	8s R	9s R	10s R	7s r	8s r	9s r	10s r
2 Dynamic Webbing Curl	Team 1	1 Pad/2 Pads	8-12 pulls 55% of RM	8-12 pulls 60% of RM	8-12 pulls 65-70% of RM	8-12 pulls 70% of RM	4-6 pulls 75-80% of RM	4-6 pulls 80-85% of RM	4-6 pulls 85-90% of RM	4-6 pulls 90-95% of RM	4-6 pulls 75-80% of RM	4-6 pulls 80-85% of RM	4-6 pulls 85-90% of RM	4-6 pulls 90-95% of RM
	Team 2	1 Pad/2 Pads	8-12 pulls 55% of RM	8-12 pulls 60% of RM	8-12 pulls 65-70% of RM	8-12 pulls 70% of RM	4-6 pulls 75-80% of RM	4-6 pulls 80-85% of RM	4-6 pulls 85-90% of RM	4-6 pulls 90-95% of RM	4-6 pulls 75-80% of RM	4-6 pulls 80-85% of RM	4-6 pulls 85-90% of RM	4-6 pulls 90-95% of RM
	Team 3	1 Pad/2 Pads	8-12 pulls 55% of RM	8-12 pulls 60% of RM	8-12 pulls 65-70% of RM	8-12 pulls 70% of RM	4-6 pulls 75-80% of RM	4-6 pulls 80-85% of RM	4-6 pulls 85-90% of RM	4-6 pulls 90-95% of RM	4-6 pulls 75-80% of RM	4-6 pulls 80-85% of RM	4-6 pulls 85-90% of RM	4-6 pulls 90-95% of RM
	1 Finger	1 Pad/2 Pads	8-12 pulls 55% of RM	8-12 pulls 60% of RM	8-12 pulls 65-70% of RM	8-12 pulls 70% of RM	4-6 pulls 75-80% of RM	4-6 pulls 80-85% of RM	4-6 pulls 85-90% of RM	4-6 pulls 90-95% of RM	4-6 pulls 75-80% of RM	4-6 pulls 80-85% of RM	4-6 pulls 85-90% of RM	4-6 pulls 90-95% of RM
3 Levering	Team 1	Wrap	8-12 180s	8-12 180s	8-12 180s	8-12 180s	4-6 180s	4-6 180s	4-6 180s	4-6 180s	4-6 180s	4-6 180s	4-6 180s	4-6 180s
	Team 2	Wrap	8-12 180s	8-12 180s	8-12 180s	8-12 180s	4-6 180s	4-6 180s	4-6 180s	4-6 180s	4-6 180s	4-6 180s	4-6 180s	4-6 180s
	Team 3	Wrap	8-12 180s	8-12 180s	8-12 180s	8-12 180s	4-6 180s	4-6 180s	4-6 180s	4-6 180s	4-6 180s	4-6 180s	4-6 180s	4-6 180s
	1 Finger	Wrap	8-12 180s	8-12 180s	8-12 180s	8-12 180s	4-6 180s	4-6 180s	4-6 180s	4-6 180s	4-6 180s	4-6 180s	4-6 180s	4-6 180s

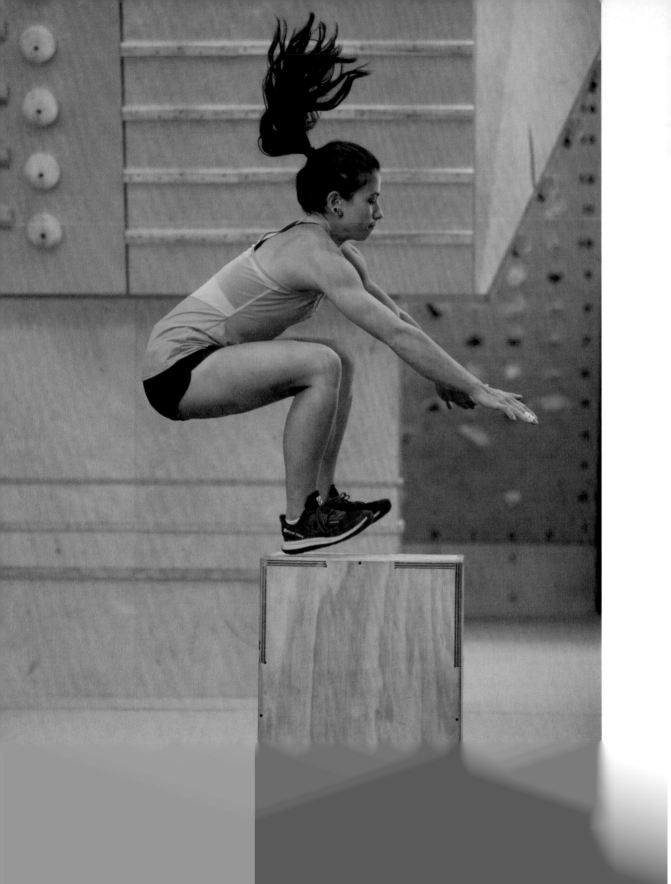

Chapter 5

OFF-THE-WALL FITNESS

THE MORE YOU PROGRESS AS A CLIMBER, the fitter you will be—including having more muscle and less fat on your frame. Beyond spending time on the wall and using the specialized training tools featured in the Climbing Supplements chapter, the weight room is the often-overlooked climber's best friend. You might have started climbing for an alternative upper body workout because you found the weight room boring and tedious, which is understandable, but the best part about weight training specifically for climbing is that you know everything you do will directly benefit you on the wall. It's an efficient and effective way to strengthen crucial climbing muscles.

If you're looking for a boost in climbing performance, one of the following workouts could be just what you need. Some yoga poses are particularly good for tightly muscled climbers who need to increase flexibility. The most important muscle groups, and why they matter to climbers, are described. Each workout includes explanations of the individual exercises, as well as how to combine them all together in one session to maximize results. Consider adding one to two of these workouts every week. You can do them on a non-climbing day or after a climbing session— just make sure to save some energy.

CORE

Fingers of steel, strong arms and legs, and mental focus are useless without a solid core to link it all together.

The "core" consists of the midsection, from the abs and obliques (side abdominals) to the mid and lower back and hips. There are dozens of smaller muscles that make up the "core," and they all perform as one unit to link the different parts of the upper and lower body. Your core wraps around your torso and supports everything, making separate movements in your limbs and torso work together for one common goal. There's not a single thing in climbing (or life, really) that doesn't involve the core, and strengthening it is invaluable for preventing injury, especially to the lower back and shoulders. This area of the body builds strength quickly, but remember to work all the muscles that comprise it.

BICEPS

Welcome to the gun show. Biceps coordinate the complicated and intricate movements of the hand, as well as flex and rotate the forearms. Without the biceps, you wouldn't be able to bend your arms at the elbow or twist your hands in the strange ways climbing demands. These muscles are also particularly important for lockoffs and underclings.

FOREARMS

Sinewy, vein-popping forearms are a dead giveaway that you're a hardcore climber. Our sport's never-ending demands on this group of relatively small muscles build them up into freakishly jacked and vascular tools. The forearms are the operating force behind pinches, crimps, gastons, underclings, and more. Although they are usually the first body part to give out when climbing (the dreaded pump), they are also some of the quickest muscles to develop when training.

BACK

Climbing is all about pulling, and the back has the biggest and strongest "pull" muscle group in the body. The latissimus dorsi (lats), rhomboid, and trapezius (traps) are the three large muscles responsible for every climber's ability to pull. As a result of frequent climbing, the upper back can overdevelop to give you a "hunchback" appearance, even if a person doesn't do a single pull-up or other back exercise.

LEGS

Though your legs are the foundation of your strength, they are easily overlooked when training. As the most underrated cog in the machine, the legs are literally the driving force behind most movement. Your upper body holds you onto the wall, but your legs propel you upward. Because these muscles are so large (compared to the smaller arm muscles), aim to use them as much and as efficiently as possible. Calves are crucial for kneebars and for standing on dime edges, pockets, and smears, while quads are the secret to big power moves. Hamstrings keep you on overhangs and make heel hooks and toe hooks possible.

MAKE ANY EXERCISE MORE CLIMBING SPECIFIC

Most dedicated climbers spend at least a little training time in the weight room, but much of that time is wasted performing exercises that don't mimic climbing movements closely enough. Focusing on strengthening ineffective movements can often lead to injury when climbing because you're not training the proper muscles to work in harmony. Sports science research (and basic logic) supports the theory that the more an exercise mirrors movement in the sport, the more the exercise positively affects performance. For climbing, the secret to a successful training exercise session off the wall is to maintain a body position common to climbing. Six basic rules can be applied to standard exercises to make them more climbing-specific. By making these small modifications and paying careful attention to your body, from your big toe to your fingertips, you can drastically increase the effectiveness of almost any exercise, whether you're lifting heavy dumbbells or using your own body weight.

The Workout

The following rules were created by studying the most ideal climbing posture. This posture varies by terrain, angle, hold type, etc., but you'll find these suggestions reflect the most often-used postures. Some of these rules may seem intuitive, especially to more advanced climbers, but think about the last time you went into the weight room—you might not have employed any of these. The more rules you can incorporate into any one exercise, the more beneficial your non-climbing training time will be. This even helps train your mind to activate several different body parts simultaneously, which makes you a more fluid and intuitive climber. Simply

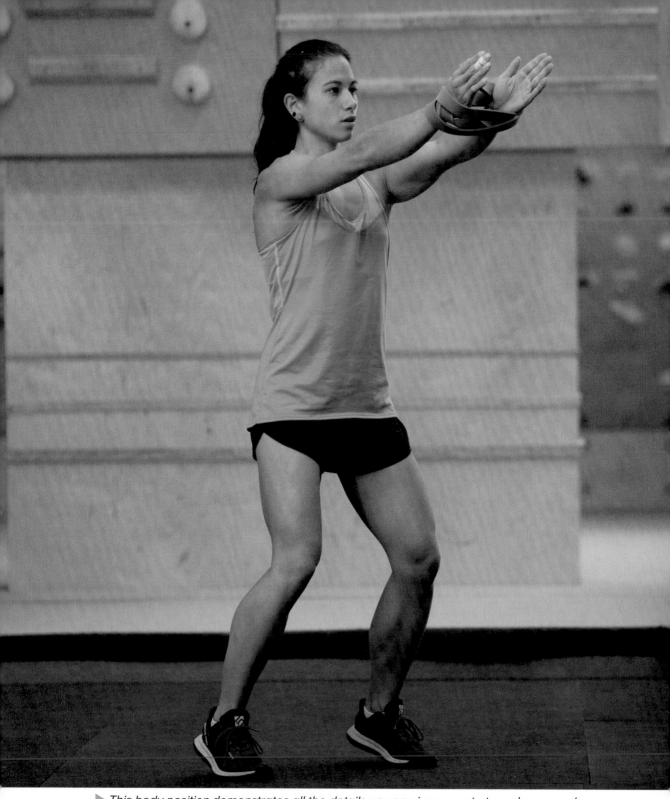

▶ *This body position demonstrates all the details you can incorporate to make general exercises more climbing specific.*

put, for maximum benefit and injury prevention, make your weight room exercises mirror climbing.

The Rules

▶ **Weight Toes**: When climbing, you rarely ever transfer your full weight into your heels. Your toes do almost all the work to power your legs and balance over holds. So when training for climbing, it is important to shift your weight into your toes. Don't stand all the way up on your tippy toes, but think about shifting your weight forward onto the ball of your foot and slightly elevating your heel; this is how you spend 99 percent of your climbing time—and probably 0 percent of training time off the wall. It's best applied to exercises that normally focus on the upper body—bicep curls, shoulder presses, bent-over rows—because most lower body exercises already have a recommended stance. Build up endurance by doing simple calf raises, with or without weight, then try to do them one leg at a time to mimic climbing movement even more closely. If that is too easy, try performing a flag maneuver (one leg kicked out to the side, behind the other) while doing raises, or close your eyes to add more of a balance challenge.

▶ **Bend Knees**: Every beginning climber is told to straighten his arms so he hangs on his skeleton instead of using up precious biceps and forearm energy. But to straighten your arms, you must bend your knees. This transfers weight from the arms to the stronger legs, where your body's most powerful muscles are designed to support and transfer your entire weight easily and efficiently. With that in mind, do exercises that train your knees to bend while your arms simultaneously reach or pull. Performing arm-centric exercises like triceps extensions in a squat position, rather than standing upright, teaches your leg muscles to engage during arm movement. Building this muscle-activation memory helps every aspect of your climbing tremendously.

▶ **Engage Abdominals**: Maintaining core tension allows for effective transfer of energy from your feet to your hands. In addition, the more stable your midsection, the more efficient your movement. The core muscles are rarely used to initiate a move, so stay away from exercises, such as standard crunches, that don't resemble climbing. Instead, focus more on exercises that keep a stable midsection while performing arm or leg movements, like performing a high plank

Game: All the Grades

Number of Players

1+

Setup

Pick a grade at least a number or two below your onsight level.

How to Play

Climb all problems or routes of that particular grade in the gym, whether boulders, topropes, or lead climbs.

Training Purpose

Endurance, onsight ability, technique

Game: Beta Games

Number of Players

2+

Setup

Have one person climb a problem, and pay close attention to her exact beta.

How to Play

Climb the problem exactly like your friend, using every move. Choose differing styles to add variety.

Training Purpose

Working weaknesses, conscientious movement, experimenting with beta

while lifting one arm or leg at a time. Try to keep your midsection still while moving the chosen limb in a controlled fashion, which is exactly what you should try to achieve while climbing.

▶ **Retract Shoulder Blades**: The shoulder blades provide the stable foundation for your mobile arms. When you engage your shoulder blades down your back, you can take stress and weight off your arms and shoulders, helping to direct the force into your midsection. To demonstrate this, raise a weight above your head with your shoulder blades relaxed and shoulders slumped forward, then lift the same weight with your shoulder blades retracted. Which is easier? You will notice the weight feels much lighter in the latter case. When you engage your large shoulder blade muscles, you give additional support to your arm. Make sure to stay engaged by gently pulling them in toward your spine during all training exercises, including fingerboard training.

▶ **Keep Arms Above Shoulders**: The majority of climbing involves keeping the arms above shoulder height, though in a few instances the arms work below shoulder height (mantels, underclings, and sidepulls). Exercises with hands below the shoulders translate poorly to climbing-specific movement. Strengthen your shoulders by holding your arms out and above your shoulders and resisting against a band or strap.

▶ **Maintain Straight Elbows**: Straightening the elbows when climbing vertical and overhanging terrain puts weight onto the skeleton and takes it out of the shoulder muscles and biceps. This allows for greater circulation and more energy-efficient movement. Unless you're focusing on lockoff strength with bicep-bending movements, try to keep your arms straight during other exercises, such as arm circles and straight-arm raises.

COMPLETE CORE

A strong core is crucial to being physically fit and strong, especially in climbing. Body tension, keeping your feet on, moving efficiently, toeing-in on overhangs—they all revolve around the core. Plus, a solid core helps prevent injury. Many core workouts in the past focused solely on the front abdominals, which is only one part of a complex muscle system. It's important to work all the muscles in your trunk: front, back, side, and all the tiny stabilizers in between. The following varied exercises are specifically targeted to work multiple parts of your body at the same time—just like climbing does.

The Workout

Pick five or more of these exercises and do them at least three (and up to five) times a week for best results. Add as many sets or exercises as you need to feel the burn; you should be struggling to complete the last set. Do these any time—at the end of a climbing session, on a rest day, in the morning before work—except for right before you climb, as this could wear out your core and give you poor, injury-causing technique. Each of these exercises has varied motions to work your front, back, and sides. Take at least one to two rest days from core work every week to let your muscles recover. If you have a history of back or neck problems, consult your doctor before starting high-intensity exercises like these.

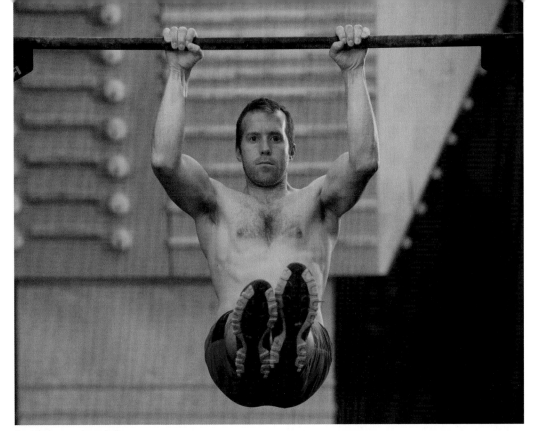

▶ *Hanging Leg Lift*

The Exercises

Hanging Leg Lift: Start on the jugs of a hangboard or on a pull-up bar. Keep your arms straight, shoulders engaged (squeeze shoulder blades together), and legs straight down. Lift your legs so your hips are at 90 degrees, without bending your knees. When you lower back down, keep your body as still as possible (you'll have a tendency to swing). Raise your legs again without using momentum. Do three sets of fifteen, resting about one minute between sets.

▶ **Variation**: For a tougher challenge, raise your legs with knees bent, pulling them all the way into your chest. Or try just hanging with knees bent, hips at 90 degrees, and have a friend put weight on your lap. Start with 10 to 15 pounds, hanging for fifteen seconds. Have your friend remove the weight before you lower your legs.

▶ **Focus:** Abs, lower back, hip flexors

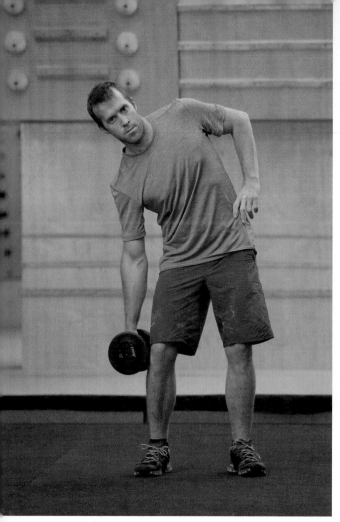 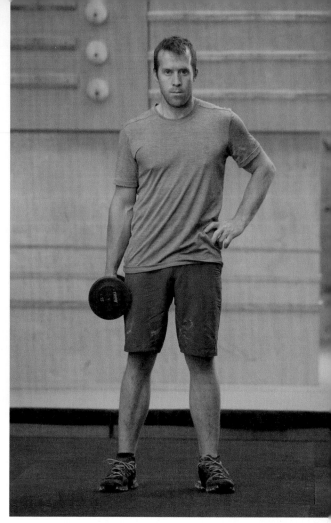

▶ *Arm Dip*

Arm Dip: Stand straight, feet shoulder-distance apart. Choose a dumbbell that will provide good resistance; 15 pounds is a good starting point. Hold it in your right hand and slowly lower your right shoulder straight down, as far as it will go. Try to keep your right hip in line with your body; don't let it jut out to the side. In a controlled motion, bring the weight and your body back up to the starting position. The up and the down should be two separate motions. Do twenty reps and then switch arms.

   ▶ **Focus**: Obliques

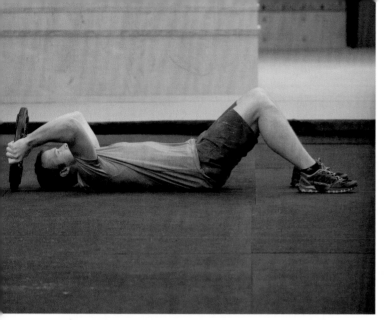

▶ *Lie on the floor like you're about to do a sit-up.*

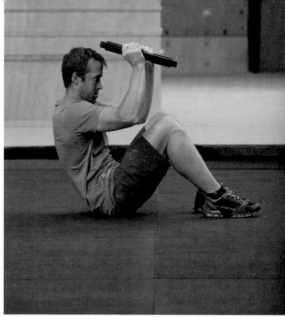

▶ *Squeeze your abs to sit all the way up.*

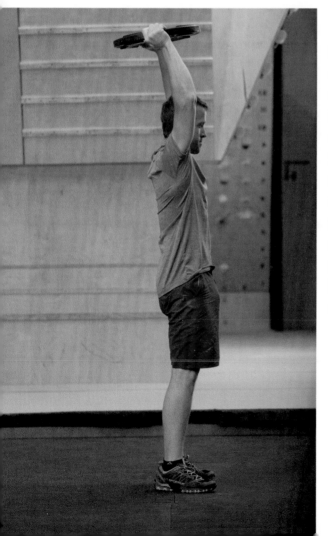

Sit Up, Stand Up: Lie supine, knees bent, feet on the floor. With your arms straight out over your head, hold a weight plate (start with 20 pounds) near the ground. Using momentum, do a sit-up with the plate in the air, get your feet under you near your butt, and stand up all the way—keeping the plate in the air. Lie back down in the starting position (plate doesn't have to be up when sitting back down, but don't put it on the ground); repeat fifteen times.

▶ **Focus:** Abs, hip flexors, hamstrings, quads, shoulders

▶ *Use your whole body to stand up with weight held above your head.*

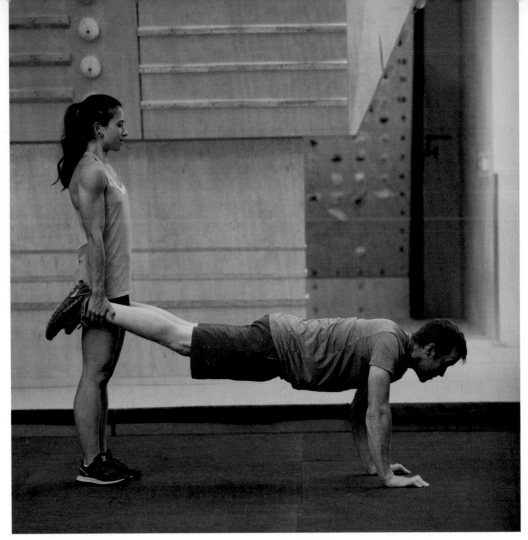

▶ *Wheelbarrow Walk*

Wheelbarrow Walk: Those wheelbarrow races you did as a kid are actually great for your core. Get into a high plank, with your hands directly below your shoulders. Have a partner lift you by your ankles. Keeping your body straight (don't dip at the waist) and looking straight ahead, move your right hand forward about 6 inches. Then move your left hand 6 inches past your right, finding a good pace for you and your partner to avoid face planting. Keep your core and glutes contracted to maximize the movement. Go about 30 feet, then switch with your partner. Try to do five rounds, without compromising technique.

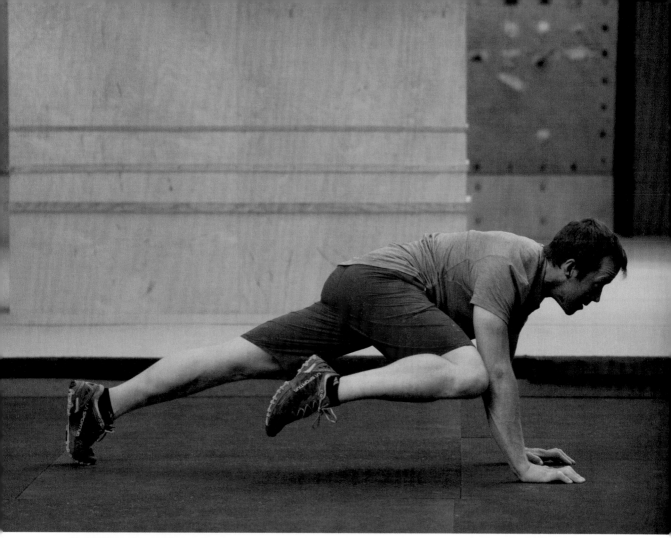

▶ *Oblique Knee-Raise Plank*

▶ **Focus:** Obliques, abs, lower back, glutes, shoulders, arms

Oblique Knee-Raise Plank: Start in a high plank. Bend one leg and bring your knee to just outside the corresponding elbow. This should open your groin up to the ground as you move your knee up. Return to starting position and repeat with the other leg. Keep it controlled but maintain a steady pace. Do this for one minute.

▶ **Focus:** Abs, lower back, obliques, glutes, hip flexors, shoulders, chest

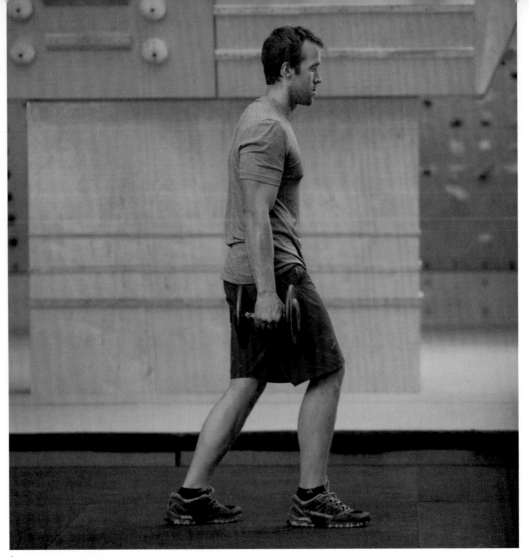

▶ *Farmer's Walk*

Farmer's Walk: Pick two weights in the high end of your comfort range. Holding one in each hand, start walking. For this motion to be effective, keep your core tight and your posture straight, standing as tall as you can. Either go for distance (50 yards) or time (1 minute). If you want to test yourself, walk until your arms are about to give out; just be careful not to drop the weights.

▶ **Variation**: Instead of using the same weight in each hand, hold a weight that's about five pounds heavier in one hand. This will force you to keep your core tight as you try to compensate for the two different weights.

▶ **Focus**: Lower back, obliques, abs, forearms, hamstrings, quads, calves

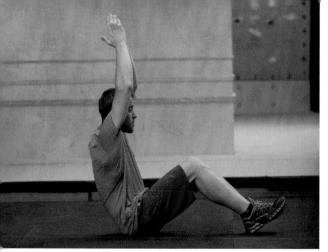 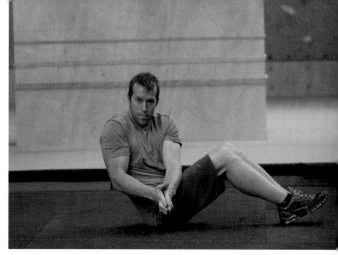

▶ *A-Frame Arm Drop*

A-Frame Arm Drop: Begin in a C-sit position, knees bent at 90 degrees, abs engaged so the upper body is off the floor, with only your heels on the ground. Put both arms straight above your head, holding palms together. While keeping your upper and lower body completely still, slowly lower your arms down to the right of your hip, tap the floor, and bring them back up overhead. Now lower to the left side. Do thirty total, fifteen per side.

▶ **Focus**: Abs, obliques, lower back, shoulders

Plank Variations: With the full-body burn they create, it's hard to ignore planks as an effective core-strengthening exercise, though they can be tedious. Here, however, are a few variations to keep them interesting. For each, keep muscles engaged and actively holding the plank. Start with three rounds of one minute, resting one minute between rounds.

▶ **Elevated plank**: This is a standard high plank, but you want your toes up on an elevated surface (bench, chair, etc.), so that your whole body is parallel to the floor. Use a wobbly exercise ball for increased difficulty.

▶ **Sideways-walking plank**: Get into high-plank position. From here, move your right hand about 6 inches to the right, and then move your left hand 6 inches right. Move your left hand back to starting position and follow with your right. Go to the left side, then repeat.

▶ **Side plank with leg raise**: In a side-plank position (left hand on floor directly under shoulder, body straight, balancing on outside edge of left foot), raise the right leg so your feet are wider than your shoulders, and hold.

▶ **Focus**: Full body

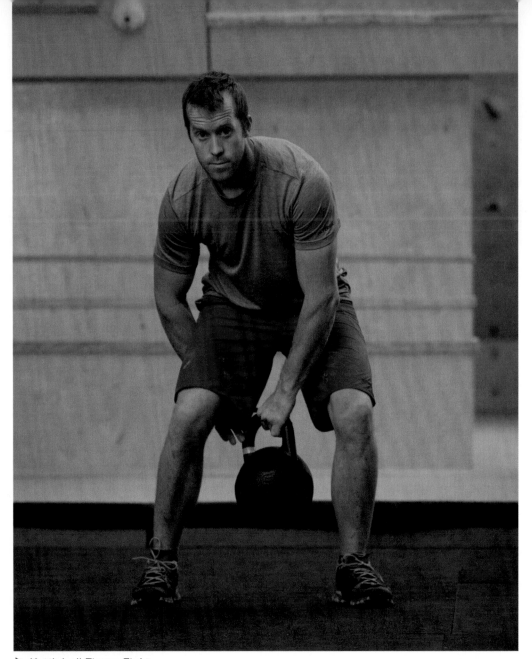

▶ *Kettlebell Figure Eight*

Kettlebell Figure Eight: Start with your legs a little wider than shoulder width, and bend at the waist, keeping your back flat and head up. Use a lightweight kettlebell, and go around your right leg with your right hand, then pass it under your right leg to your left hand. Repeat on the left side. That's one rep; repeat fifteen times.

▶ **Focus:** Abs, lower back, glutes, hip flexors, obliques, arms, quads

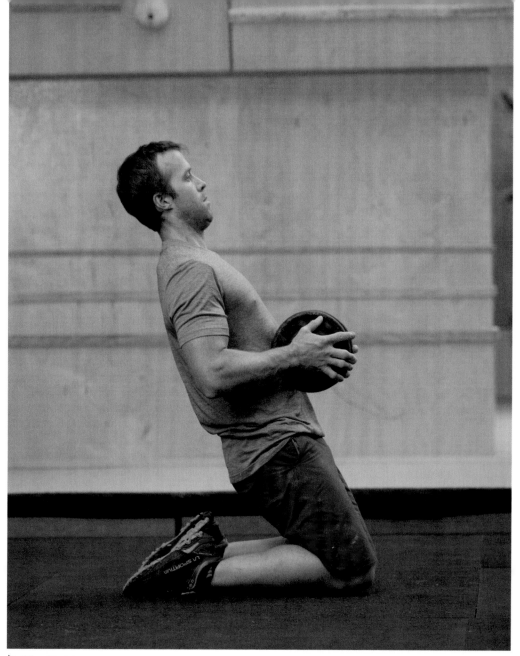

▶ *The Matrix*

The Matrix: Start on your knees, hip-width apart, with a straight back. Hold a weight near your belly button and slowly lean back as far as you can, keeping your back straight. Hold for three seconds, and then slowly come back to the starting position. Repeat twenty times.

▶ **Focus**: Abs, lower back, glutes, quads, hip flexors

DO THE LEGWORK

Many climbers can quickly rattle off a number of excuses for skipping leg day in the weight room—"My legs will get too bulky and weigh me down" and "This couch is too comfortable to leave" are favorites—but there are plenty of reasons to focus on strengthening your legs. Having a strong, powerful, and flexible lower half gives you more endurance, allows you to do bigger, harder moves, and exponentially improves footwork, and thus technique. Sport climbers need sturdy calves and hamstrings to really toe-in on the steeps, and boulderers need a powerful range of motion to make big, dynamic moves. With any type of climbing, the more weight you can put on your feet and legs, the longer your comparatively weaker arms and upper body will last. Here is a collection of quick and simple exercises to build your base and make you a better climber.

The Workout

These exercises can be done with no weight (aim for high reps or a good chunk of time), but three sets of ten reps with a challenging but doable weight will build strength quickly. If using weights, pick something that's about 70 percent of your max. Do these once per week on a non-climbing day, or on a day when you're only doing light or easy climbing.

The Exercises

Squats and Deadlifts: No matter your pursuit, the squat and the deadlift are the two most fundamental and comprehensive lower body exercises for athletes. Each works every muscle from your calves to your glutes to your core, and both are important for all types of movement. If you only have a few minutes, focus on doing squats and deadlifts.

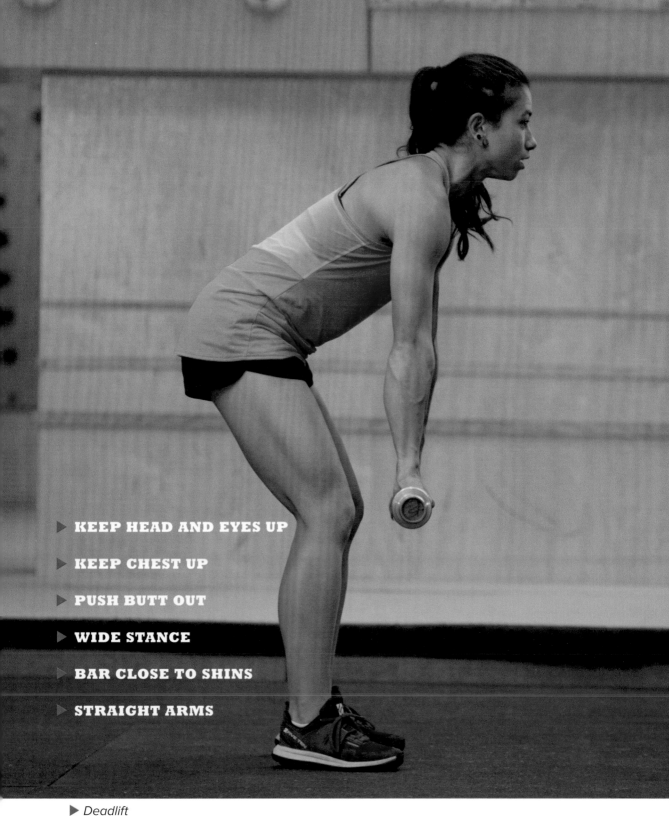

▶ KEEP HEAD AND EYES UP

▶ KEEP CHEST UP

▶ PUSH BUTT OUT

▶ WIDE STANCE

▶ BAR CLOSE TO SHINS

▶ STRAIGHT ARMS

▶ *Deadlift*

Toeing In: Increase calf and toe strength to make use of the smallest nubbins on overhangs, and to improve balance and stability for delicate, techy moves on slabby and vertical terrain. For each of the listed exercises, aim for high reps (fifty-plus) when unweighted, three sets of ten when weighted, or time (thirty to forty-five seconds as a starting point).

▶ **Catcher calf raises**: Bend down into a baseball catcher's position, knees pointed slightly outward. Raise heels up and down in a smooth, fluid motion. Make it easier by using one hand on the ground (for balance only), or make it harder by holding a light dumbbell or kettlebell at your chest.

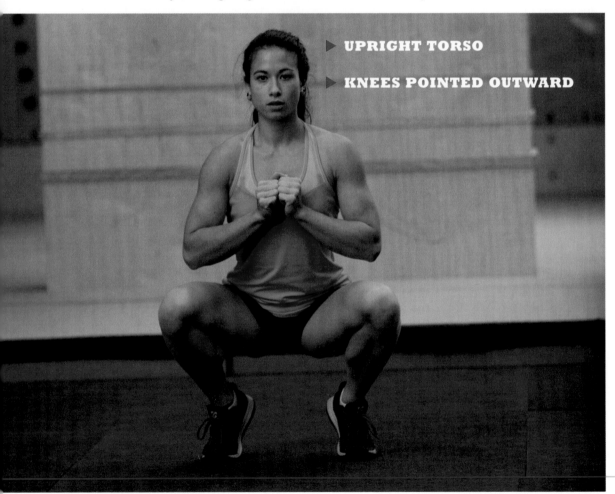

▶ UPRIGHT TORSO

▶ KNEES POINTED OUTWARD

▶ *Catcher Calf Raises*

▶ **Calf raises**: Find a curb or stair, or stack a couple of weight plates on the ground. The balls of the feet should be on the lift with the back half of the feet hanging off. Drop your feet to feel a stretch in the calf, and then press up through your toes till you're on your tip-toes. Hold weight for a strength challenge, or do one leg at a time to focus on balance.

▶ **Continuous calf jumps**: On flat ground, jump up and down using just your toes; bend your knees only slightly and don't let your heels touch the ground.

High Stepping: This move requires a combination of balance and flexibility, along with strength throughout the entire range of motion. Aim for three sets of fifteen for each leg.

▶ **Weighted box steps**: Find a box or ledge at shin height and step up with the left leg, bring the right up, step down with the left leg first, then follow with the right. Repeat by stepping up first with the right leg. Make sure to put your whole foot on the box. Add weight, include a calf raise at the top of the step, or find a higher box for a greater challenge.

▶ **Bulgarian lunges**: Using a bench placed behind you, extend one leg backward and place the top of the foot so it's resting on the flat surface (rest on just the toes to make it slightly harder). With a dumbbell in each hand, lunge forward until your front knee reaches 90 degrees, being careful that it doesn't extend past your toes. Lunge with the front leg farther away from the bench (the rear leg will be straighter) to increase the difficulty.

▶ **Hanging knee lifts**: This is a core-intensive exercise, but it's excellent for hip flexor strength and overall flexibility. Hang from a bar and raise one or both knees toward your chest, going as high as possible. Alternate between keeping your knees together and spreading them wide for increased range of motion.

Stemming: Requiring endurance, flexibility, and some serious calf strength, stemming utilizes the rarely used outer muscles of the hips to help push outward against the wall. Go for time (one minute) or a high number of reps; you should feel the burn for the last few reps/seconds. Use weight for increased difficulty.

▶ **Wall sits**: These are ideal for pushing through the burn in a safe position while building leg endurance and mental fortitude. Find a wall and "sit" with your back against it and legs at 90 degrees. Place a lightweight plate on top of your thighs to up the challenge. Keep palms flat on the wall next to you, or rest them lightly in your lap—don't cheat by pushing on your legs or the wall!

▶ **Multidirectional lunges:** Start standing. Keeping the core tight and the upper body upright, step forward into a lunge, then go back to the start. With the same leg, step out at about 45 degrees, then back to the start. Next step out straight to the side, then back to the start. Repeat with the other leg.

▶ **Core-to-toe side lunges**: From a standing position, lunge out to the right, keeping toes pointed forward and the left leg completely straight. Get as deep into the lunge as you can, then spring back up to standing and, without resting your right leg on the ground, lift it up as high as you can out to the side, keeping it as straight as possible. Do this without weight at first, working to make the step out of the lunge and leg lift as fluid and powerful as possible.

UPPER BODY TABATA

Climbing demands power and endurance: Power to make it through cruxes, and endurance to hang on during the easier climbing between those cruxes. With Tabata interval training, you can strengthen both power and endurance via a few focused minutes in a brutal but effective workout. So, what are Tabatas? In 1997, Dr. Izumi Tabata developed a method that challenges the body's aerobic and anaerobic energy pathways by forcing the muscles to fire when they're locked up with lactic acid (i.e., totally pumped).

The Workouts

Power Flush: A Tabata interval lasts two minutes per individual exercise; you should perform it twice weekly for maximum effectiveness. When choosing a weight, use about 60 percent of your one-rep max (e.g., if you can curl 50 pounds with both arms once only, then your Tabata weight would be 30 pounds). For twenty seconds at a time, and working toward a maximum number of reps, perform each exercise in bulk, resting ten seconds between intervals. Do each exercise for 20 seconds, rest 10 seconds, work 20 seconds, rest 10 seconds, and so on until you've done two minutes of one exercise. Rest two minutes before repeating the 20 on/10 off with the next exercise. Continue until you've done all four exercises. The number of reps may decrease during each successive round, but stick with the time (use a stopwatch), giving maximum effort with controlled, rapid movement. After a few sessions, you should see your total number of reps increasing—tangible evidence that your ability to clear lactic acid (i.e., delay the pump) has improved. Note that the following four exercises focus on climbing-specific muscles, working the large muscle groups first and ending with the smallest.

Once you've increased conditioning, work your way up to four minutes for each individual exercise, called "16 Minutes of Hell." You'll do the same 20 on/10 off cycle seven times for each exercise, resting two minutes between each movement.

The Exercises

Bent row: Grab a dumbbell in each hand and bend forward at the waist, such that your torso is at nearly 90 degrees to the lower body; your knees should be slightly bent. Let the weight hang. Keep your back straight and stomach tight. Pull the weight as far as possible toward your armpit, aiming for a spot right alongside the chest. Extend your arms back toward the ground with intent.

Lat pulldown: This exercise requires a cable machine. Grasp a cable bar with a wide grip and tuck your thighs under the supports. Pull the bar toward your chest until it touches your sternum. Let the bar return upward until your arms are extended.

Biceps curl: Grab a dumbbell in each hand. Start with your arms straight and your elbows close to your sides. Raise both dumbbells simultaneously, bringing the weights all the way up to your shoulders. Lower until your arms are straight.

Wrist curls: Sit and grasp a barbell with a narrow to shoulder-width underhand grip (palms facing up). Rest your forearms on your thighs with your wrists extending just past your knees. Let the barbell roll from the palm down to the fingers, then grab the barbell and curl your wrist back toward you.

SUSPENDED CIRCUITS

The TRX (total resistance exercise) suspension trainer utilizes two adjustable straps with handles in creative configurations to use your body weight for resistance. Many climbing gyms have TRX straps or adjustable gymnastic rings that can be used the same way. Suspension training engages those tiny stabilizing muscles in your core, shoulders, legs, and back that are necessary for climbing but often not addressed by traditional weight machines and dumbbell exercises. The following is a fifteen-minute circuit of exercises that strengthens your core and stabilizes your shoulders to eliminate weak spots in your overall fitness.

The Workout

Do this twice a week, on rest days. Aim to complete each exercise at least once, though you can do up to three sets of each exercise. Transition and rest thirty seconds between each exercise and two minutes between each round or circuit. "Mid-calf" means stirrups should come to mid-calf. "Long" is slightly longer than that; "short" is shorter.

Circuit 1

Core Round 1. Targeting core stability and strength, all of these workouts directly translate to better performance on steep sections, where body tension, deliberate foot placement, and staying close to the wall are crucial.

▶ **Body Saw**. 8 reps; mid-calf length

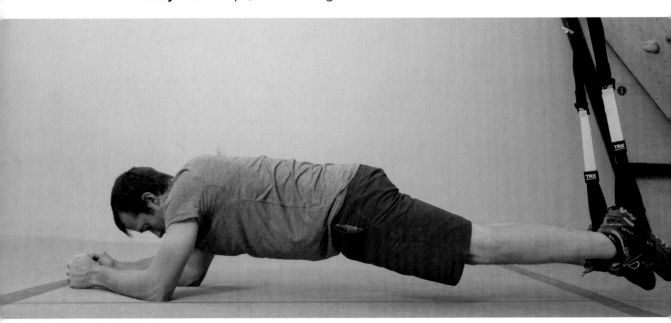

▶ *TRX Body Saw*

In forearm plank position (toes flexed downward in stirrups), place your elbows under your shoulders. Slowly push your body as far forward as possible, and then backward to complete one rep. Don't let your hips sag. To increase difficulty, try the workout with hands on the floor and straight arms.

▶ **Helps with**: Body control while moving, high stepping, staying tight on overhangs, preventing barn doors

▶ **Side Plank with Hip Raise**. 8 reps (per side); mid-calf length

Start in a push-up position, then turn into side plank position (elbow under shoulder and top arm straight toward sky). Place your feet in stirrups with the top foot in front, heel to toe. With straight legs, raise your hips slightly, then return to starting position for one rep.

▶ **Helps with**: Drop-knees, cutting feet, high heel hooks

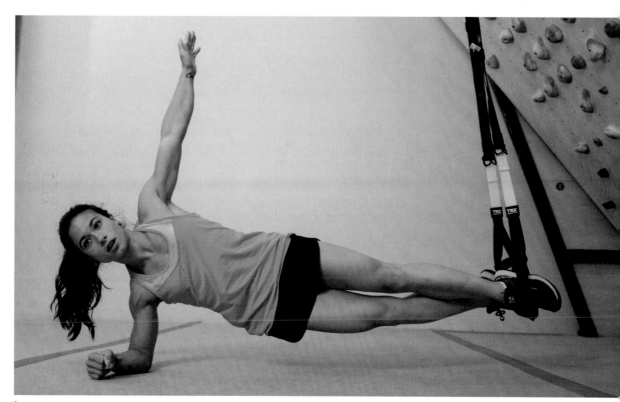

▶ *TRX Side Plank with Hip Raise*

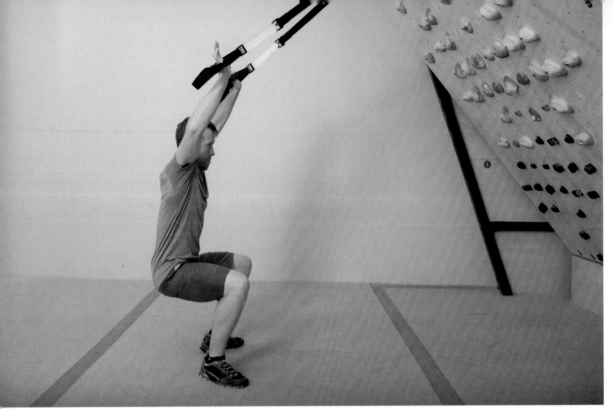

▶ *TRX Overhead Squat*

▶ **Overhead Squat**. 8 reps; mid-calf length

Stand with your feet shoulder-width apart, facing the anchor point. Place your hands inside the stirrups with the backs of your hands against the straps, thumbs on the outside. Raise your hands above your head, wider than your shoulders. Without leaning, squeeze your upper back to put tension on the straps. Maintain this tension with your chest forward and eyes up, then squat as low as you can. In the bottom of the squat, squeeze shoulders and back for more tension, then stand up for one rep.

▶ **Helps with**: Preventing hunchback, opening chest, hip strength and flexibility for steeps, body tension

Circuit 2

Shoulder Stability. These exercises isolate and strengthen the entire shoulder girdle, which is prone to injury in climbers, by putting the shoulder in climbing-specific positions. It also builds strength and flexibility throughout the upper back.

▶ **Clock Press**. 3 reps; long adjustment

With heels up, lean into the stirrups in a low-angle push-up position. Lower your chest to your hands, then slowly extend one arm out to the side, pause, and bring it back. Repeat with the opposite arm, then push back to the start for one rep. Go closer to the ground to make it harder.

  ▶ **Helps with**: Compression, sidepulls, preventing shoulder injuries

▶ **Deltoid Series: T to Y to I**. 8 reps; long adjustment

Put one foot in front of the other, with your arms in front holding straps. For "T," stand up by putting your arms out to the sides, shifting weight from back to front, and squeezing your shoulder blades. Lower back down, then repeat in "Y," lower, then arms straight up for "I"; that's one rep.

  ▶ **Helps with**: Overhanging shoulder-specific moves, gastons, sidepulls, compression

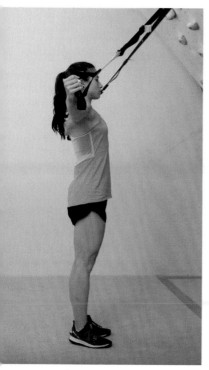 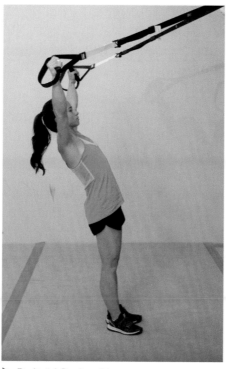 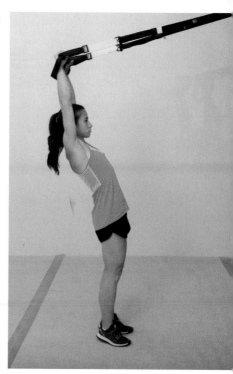

▶ *Deltoid Series: T*   ▶ *Deltoid Series: Y*   ▶ *Deltoid Series: I*

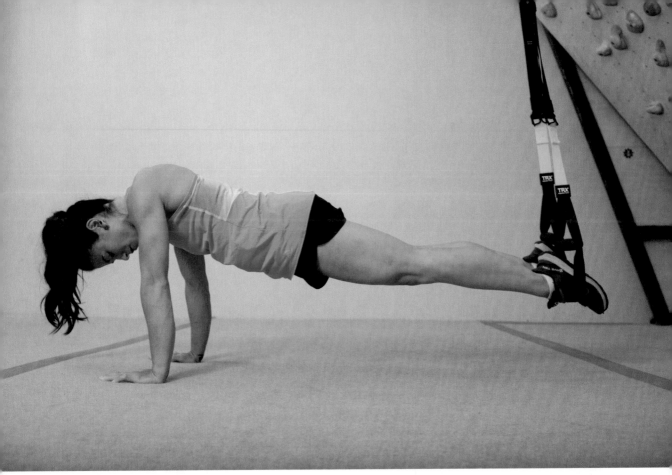

▶ *TRX Atomic Push-up Matrix*

▶ **Atomic Push-up Matrix**. 8 reps; mid-calf length

In a push-up position with your feet in stirrups, bring your knees into your left elbow with slight rotation, return to the start, then bring your knees into your right elbow and go back to start. Bring your knees straight up to your chest, go back to start, and then do a push-up for one rep.

▶ **Helps with**: High foot placement and heel hooks, body tension, strengthening opposition muscles, core stability

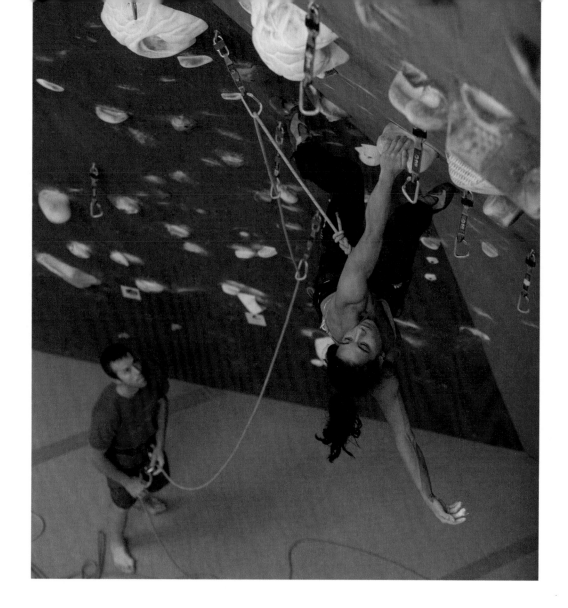

▶ **T-Spine Rotation**. 8 reps (per side); short adjustment

With your inside foot in front of the outer foot, hold the handle with your outside hand in a lockoff position, elbow high. With your inside hand parallel to straps, lower as far as possible, then extend your arm out to the side. Bring your arm back and pull yourself up to starting position. Switch feet to make it easier.

   ▶ **Helps with**: Lockoffs; hip, spine, and shoulder flexibility; controlling moves on steeps

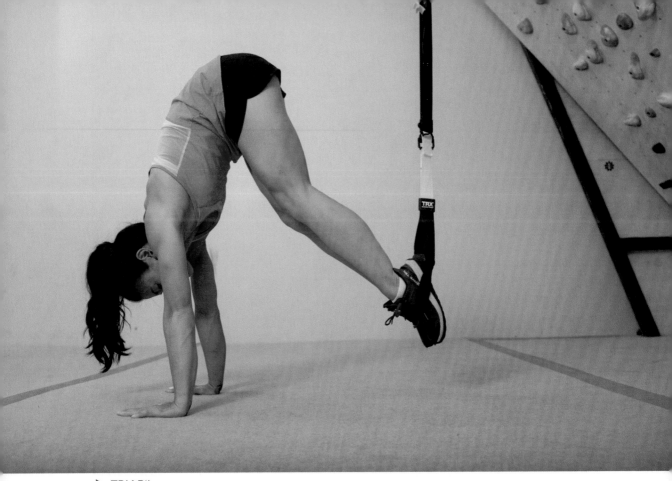

▶ *TRX Pike*

Circuit 3

Core Round 2. More isolated and advanced core exercises for keeping tension with one foot on.

▶ **Pike**. 8 reps; mid-calf length

In push-up position with your feet in stirrups, lift your tailbone up with legs straight. Lower back to starting position to complete one rep.

▶ **Helps with**: High stepping, holding a swing, body tension

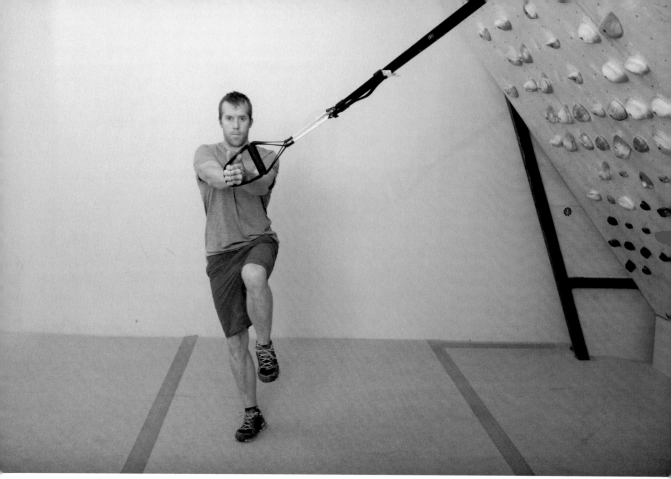

▶ *TRX Rotation Warding with March*

▶ **Rotational Warding with March**. 8 reps (per side); mid-calf length

Stand sideways with your hands in both stirrups in a prayer position. Push hard to the side with straight arms to keep straps under tension. Now slowly march by raising each knee.

▶ **Helps with**: Holding barn-door swings, core strength, body tension

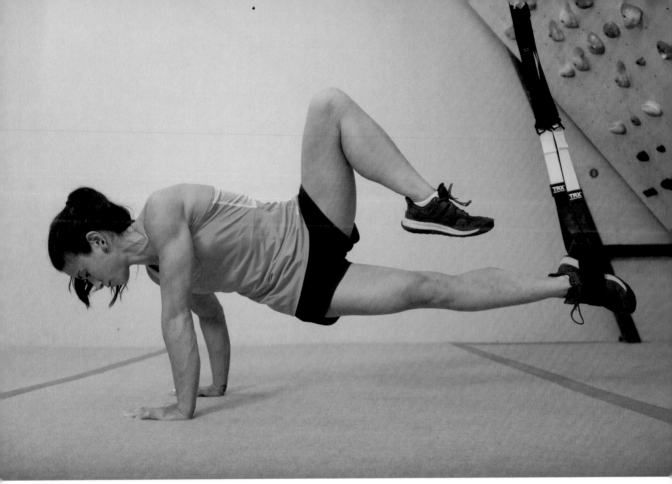

▶ *TRX Plank with Abduction and Scorpion*

▶ **Plank with Abduction and Scorpion**. 8 reps (per side); mid-calf length

In push-up position with one foot in the stirrups, bring your free knee to your chest, then back to start. Extend your leg out to the side (abduction); go back to start. Now twist at the hips to swing your leg back and over your other leg so your hips are open (scorpion). This is one rep.

▶ **Helps with**: Single-leg strength, hip flexibility, back-stepping, high stepping, body tension

STRONG CIRCUITS

If you work full-time and/or have a family, it can be difficult to squeeze in more than a few hours at the gym one night a week. What matters most in a workout is getting the most bang for your buck—this means short but intense workouts that keep you strong. The circuits listed here can keep you at or near peak performance even if you don't get to climb much. These circuits focus less on endurance, which you can easily get back with one or two endurance workouts per week, and more on strength. If possible, try to add a climbing supplement workout (campus or hangboard) at least once a week.

The Workout

Train for about forty-five minutes twice a week. Choose eight different exercises, divided into two groups of four. Within each group of four, there should be one exercise each for upper body, leg, and core, and the fourth should be an isolated pair of oppositional muscles (core/lower back, biceps/triceps, chest/upper back; choose one muscle for the first group and the other muscle for the second group). Perform each exercise for forty seconds; give yourself three seconds to switch between exercises. Complete four rounds, where in one round comprises completing all four exercises once (160 seconds of work plus transition time). Don't stop after completing each round; keep pushing until you have completed each exercise four times for a total of sixteen movements, and then rest for five minutes. Repeat these steps with the second group of movements, and then take another five-minute rest. Finish the circuit with five straight minutes of "last core" exercises.

The Exercises

The following are suggestions, but you can make up your own. To do that, closely analyze the type of moves you make while climbing (e.g., locking off, crossing through, flagging, etc.), and then integrate an established exercise that works those muscle groups. For example, if you need to do a hard pulling move on a steep roof, add in pull-ups with legs extended and hips at 90 degrees. Try to combine multiple exercises/movements to emphasize coordination, which is hugely important in climbing.

Upper Body

▶ **Mountain man**: Use a rope on a pulley hanging from the ceiling, with a climbing hold attached to each end of the rope. (Free-hanging holds like Metolius Rock Rings are excellent for this.) Pull off the ground, bringing one arm all the way down into a lockoff position, and hold for a few seconds. Then pull the other hand down and hold for a few seconds. Repeat. Increase the challenge by wearing a weight vest or using smaller holds.

▶ **Campus board touches**: Reach as high as you can with your first hand, latch the hold, and then come back to your starting position. Repeat without coming off the board. Use a foothold to make it easier, or smaller holds to make it harder.

▶ **Around the world**: Using a pull-up bar, lock off with your head just below the bar. Stay locked off and change your position by moving one hand at a time, so you're now facing the opposite direction. Continue going around the world while maintaining the lockoff; don't swing your body wildly as you swivel.

▶ **Offset pull-ups**: Throw a towel over a pull-up bar or hang a hold on it so you have something to grab that's about a foot lower than the bar itself. With one hand on the bar and the other on the towel/hold, do pull-ups. Alternate the high hand each round.

Legs

▶ **Box jumps**: Using both feet, jump onto a raised box or object; your entire foot should be on the box. Then jump back down without pausing. Repeat.

▶ **One-leg squats**: With one leg straight out in front of you, squat down on your other leg until your butt hits the heel of your foot, and then stand back up. Do this for the full forty seconds, and alternate legs each round. Use the wall for balance to make it easier or add dumbbells to make it harder.

▶ **Lunges with press**: Use a pair of light dumbbells (about 8 pounds each) and press them up straight over your head while you lunge forward. Alternate legs with each press/lunge.

▶ **Steps**: Step up onto a box or raised object, match feet, and step back off with the same leg you initiated with. Alternate legs with each step. Use a taller box or add dumbbells to increase difficulty.

Core

▶ **Paint cans**: Grab two paint cans (or something of similar height) and place them side by side on the floor about shoulder-width apart. Place your hands on the lid of each paint can and assume the push-up position. Do a push-up, tuck your legs under your body, and then extend them in front of you without touching the floor. Hold for two seconds, and then bring them back under your body and into the starting position. Repeat.

▶ **Bridge**: Lie on your back and place both feet flat on the ground, shoulder-width apart. Raise your hips as high as you can with hands on the ground, palms down, along your side. Extend one leg out or balance your feet on a stability ball for more of a challenge.

▶ **Side elbow plank**: Lie on your side, with your forearm on the floor (elbow directly below your shoulder). Lift your hips so your weight is on the outside edge of your bottom foot and your forearm/elbow. Keep hips, shoulders, legs, and feet stacked and vertically in line with your body. Alternate sides each round.

▶ **Dip-bar leg raises**: Use a dip bar to lift your body up until your arms are extended and locked. Keeping your legs straight, raise them until they are parallel to the floor. Lower them until they're at a 45-degree angle to the floor. Repeat the raise, making sure not to let your legs dangle freely. Make it easier by doing it on your elbows, or make it more difficult by holding light dumbbells between your toes.

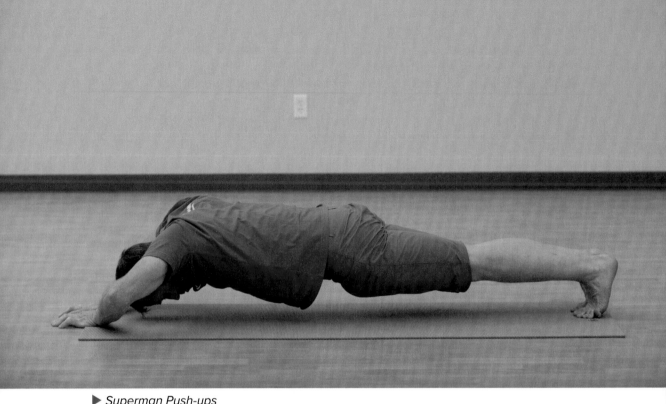

▶ *Superman Push-ups*

Oppositional

   ▶ **Core/lower back**: Crunches and Supermans (lie on your stomach with arms extended in front of you, legs shoulder-width apart; lift your arms, head, and feet straight up as high as they can go; lower slowly)

   ▶ **Biceps/triceps**: Biceps curls and overhead triceps extensions

   ▶ **Chest/upper back**: Push-ups and bent-over rows

Last Core

   ▶ **1-minute forearm plank**

   ▶ **1 minute of dolphin push-ups**: Start in a push-up position and walk your feet forward until your hips reach 90 degrees. Keep your legs straight while you do push-ups.

   ▶ **Two 30-second, one-arm planks**: Alternate arms.

▶ **1 minute of toe touches**: Lie on your back with your legs up and your hips bent at 90 degrees, heels to the ceiling; reach your hands up to touch your toes.

▶ **1 minute of scissor-kick crunches**: Lie on your back and raise your legs slightly up so your hips are bent at 30 degrees; move your left leg under your right, and then your left leg over your right while holding a crunch position with your upper body.

HOME IMPROVEMENT

Even the most diehard gym rats can't pull plastic everyday. Maybe you don't have time to get to the gym, or you're traveling and away from your routine. Whatever the reason, it's no excuse to get flabby. Here are some climbing-specific exercises you can do in a hotel room, at your house, or anywhere you have a little space and time. These movements use your own body weight (no equipment required) to improve overall cardio as well as general strength and conditioning via circuits.

The Workout

Do ten exercises back to back for one minute each, aiming for at least two rounds of ten, and resting a minimum of three minutes between each round. Add more rounds to increase difficulty. Two rounds will take less than thirty minutes, and the interval structure of working hard, then resting, will help burn fat and mimic the cardio demands of route climbing.

The Exercises

Finger hangs: Make sure the doorframe you use for this exercise is solid, and consider warming your fingers up with short hangs before going for the full set. Doorframes usually have narrow lips and should be used only if you're an intermediate or advanced climber, but tree branches or larger ledges are good alternatives. Try to keep an open-hand position. Hang five seconds then rest five seconds, repeating for the full minute.

Finger pull-ups: These should be as controlled as possible and done only after you've warmed up your fingers. Use whatever crimp position necessary (open, half-crimp, full-crimp) to do pull-ups on whatever hold or edge you have available.

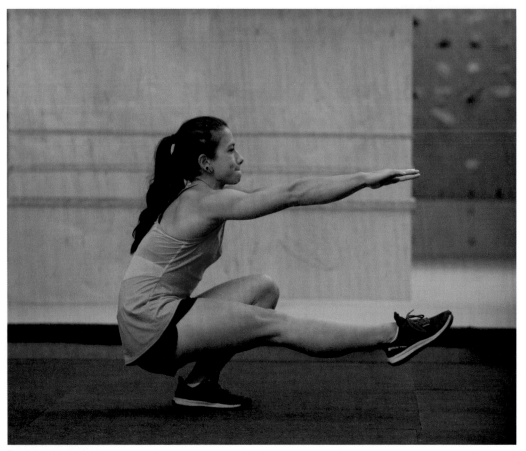

▶ *Pistol Squats*

Hanging leg raises: This is an advanced exercise that will build finger strength and work your abdominals. Hang and bring your legs up as high as possible; bend your knees to reduce difficulty or keep your legs straight for a greater challenge. Keep your core tight when lowering to prevent swinging.

Pistol squats: A pistol squat is a single-leg squat; raise one leg out in front of you and lower down as far as possible on the other leg before standing up. It's a great way to get full range of motion in each leg and build deep strength with flexibility. If you can do a full minute of pistol squats (thirty seconds per leg), great, but consider using a doorframe for assistance in getting up and down by lightly pulling on it as you come out of the squat. You can always start with regular pistol squats and finish the allotted time with assisted squats.

Side lines: Find an open space, and mark off a distance of about 100 feet with 10-foot increments. Sprint from the baseline to the end and back, reducing the distance by 10 feet on each turnaround until you are finished. Try to touch the ground at each turnaround.

Finger planks: Hold a high plank (or raised push-up position), using your fingers to hold you as high as possible. This will really build finger and core strength, as you should be fighting to stay afloat.

Raised-leg diamond push-ups: These hit the core, shoulders, triceps, chest, and back. Get into a push-up position with your hands making a diamond shape directly under your chest and raise one leg as high as possible before it bends. Perform thirty seconds of push-ups, then switch legs.

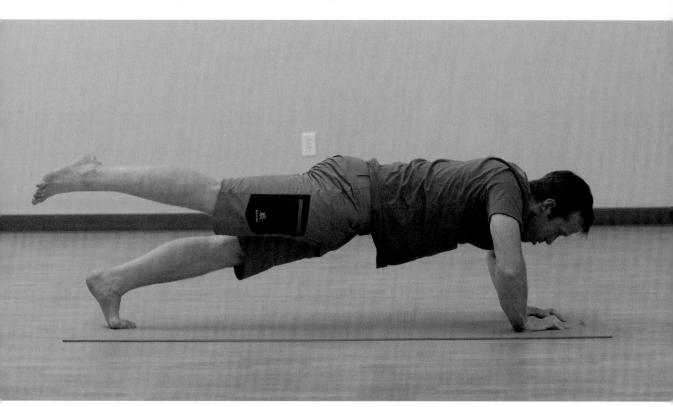

▶ *Raised-Leg Diamond Push-up*

Jumping lunges: Lower into a basic lunge, with your knee straight above your toes, not extending past them. Instead of slowly pushing back up, jump, quickly switching your legs to the alternate position while in the air, landing softly, and smoothly lowering down into the next lunge.

Superman push-ups: These will strengthen your entire core faster than anything else. Lie down in a push-up position, with hands close together and extended 10 inches out from your head. To do a push-up, you'll have to fully engage your core and bend your elbows outward.

Lateral pull-ups: Lie down under a solid table, grab the outside edge with your body straight and heels on the ground, and pull your chest to the table. The higher your feet are (closer to being level with your hands), the harder the pull-ups will be.

Upside-down shoulder press: Get into a handstand position against a wall and guide your back, glutes, and legs until you are in line vertically. Lower your body just before your head touches the ground and then press up until you are in a full handstand. Emphasize the top position with a shrug. These are great for strengthening easily injured shoulders, but make sure to warm your shoulders up with arm circles and stretching. Consider doing push-ups and/or planks first. If these are too hard, put your feet on a chair or bed with your butt in the air, hips at 90 degrees, and back straight. Now lower down—the chair or bed should take a lot of the weight off.

If you have a chair, do . . .

Triceps dips: With two chairs of the same height, put your feet on one and your upper body with straight arms on the other. Dip your upper body, keeping your back vertical, head up, and legs straight. This will emphasize shoulders, chest, triceps, and abdominals. Hold the top position for a few seconds between dips to stress abdominal burn.

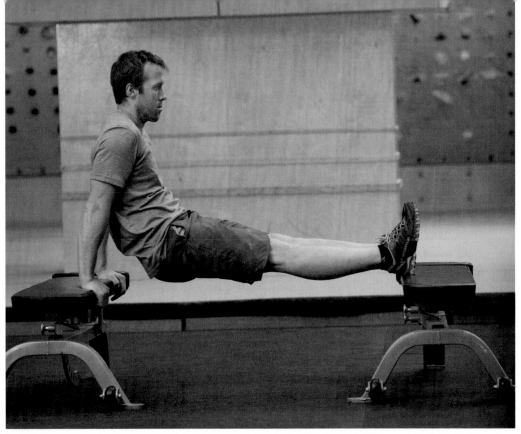

▶ Use whatever chair, bench, or machine is available for Tricep Dips.

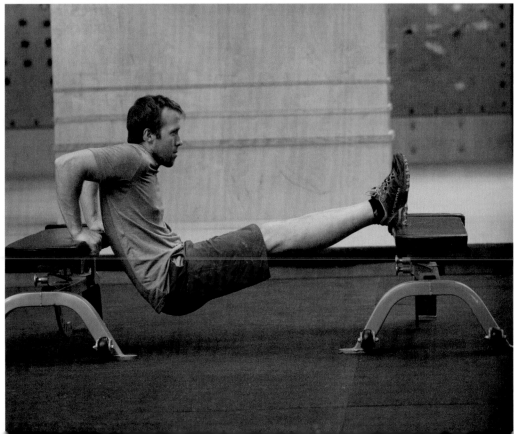

Incline push-ups: This spin on the classic push-up works your upper chest, shoulders, abdominals, and back. Place your toes on a chair or any stable, raised object, keep your back straight (don't let your butt sag), and do push-ups.

Chair-ups: These emphasizes grip and forearm strength, as well as core stability. Start by lying on your stomach (similar to Superman position) and extend your arms straight out in front of you. Grab the front legs of a chair and curl the chair upward until it's about five inches off the ground. Your elbows should always be touching the ground and are the pivot point for raising the chair. Squeeze your lats and keep your shoulders tight. You can hold the chair in the air for one minute, or choose a heavier chair and do three rounds of fifteen seconds.

If you have stairs, do . . .

Stair jumps: Similar to box jumps, except you will be jumping more forward. Find a height and distance that are optimal for you and jump forward to your desired step, landing in a squat. Jump back down and repeat. This is great for high reps and cardio. If you want to mix it up, use your momentum and consecutively leapfrog to higher steps until you reach the top of the staircase. This will test your explosiveness, stamina, and core stability.

Weighted stair walks: Just like it sounds. Find something relatively heavy that you can carry comfortably, like full water jugs, a loaded laundry basket, or a weighted pack, and walk up and down a flight of stairs. There are two things to focus on while doing these: Either go for speed with a light weight, or choose a really heavy weight and walk slowly. This can be done almost anywhere, from parking garages to apartment buildings to a nearby stadium.

Stair sprints: These will improve coordination and explosiveness. Sprint up a flight of stairs, and every round try a new pattern: each foot touches the same step; one foot on each step; skipping one step; skipping two steps; etc. Utilize your arms to help keep your momentum, and focus on the interval aspect by sprinting as hard as possible on the way up, then walking or slowly jogging down the stairs as a mini-rest.

FREAKY FIT

The following workout includes common exercises for the shoulders, legs, core, back, and arms, and many of them have a mobility component, which helps keep muscles and joints nice and loose as well.

The Workout

Do these workouts two to three times a week if you're not climbing often, or once a week when you are climbing a lot. For strength exercises: Do five sets of ten reps each of push-ups and pull-ups; do four sets of four reps for the squats and deadlifts at 80 percent of your maximum, resting one to two minutes in between. Hold the forearm plank for one minute, rest one minute, and repeat for five sets. For mobility exercises: Do five Turkish get-ups, rest one minute, and repeat for three sets. For both the plank and shoulder dislocates, do each exercise for one minute, rest one minute, and then repeat for five sets.

The Exercises

Strength

Front squat: Stand with your feet slightly wider than shoulder-width, toes pointed out about 30 to 45 degrees (but always pointing in the same direction as your knees). Rest a barbell on top of your shoulders, near your collarbones, and just touching your throat. Use a few fingers (palms up) on each hand to support the bar; your upper arm should be parallel to the floor. Inhale and slowly bend your knees, maintaining a straight spine and forward gaze. Lower all the way down until the angle between the thigh and calves is slightly less than 90 degrees (thighs are below parallel to the floor). Exhale and push up, straightening your legs and keeping your chest out and elbows up.

    Deadlift: (page 152)

    Pull-up: (page 112)

    Push-up

    Forearm plank: Start in push-up position. Bend your elbows to 90 degrees, with forearms flat on the floor and parallel to each other. (For an easier variation, interlock your fingers.) Your elbows should be directly under your shoulders, and your body should be in a straight line from your head to your heels. Keep your core tight and engaged.

Mobility

Turkish get-up: Lie on your back. Hold a kettlebell in your left hand, arm stretched straight toward the ceiling—it should stay skyward throughout the exercise. Your right leg is straight and pointing slightly away from your midline. Your right arm is on the floor, about a foot from your side. Bend your left knee, crunch up using your abs, and lean over into your right forearm. Lead with your chest—don't hunch. Transition the weight from your right forearm into your right hand. From here, push off with your left heel into a bridge with your hips off the ground. Sweep your right

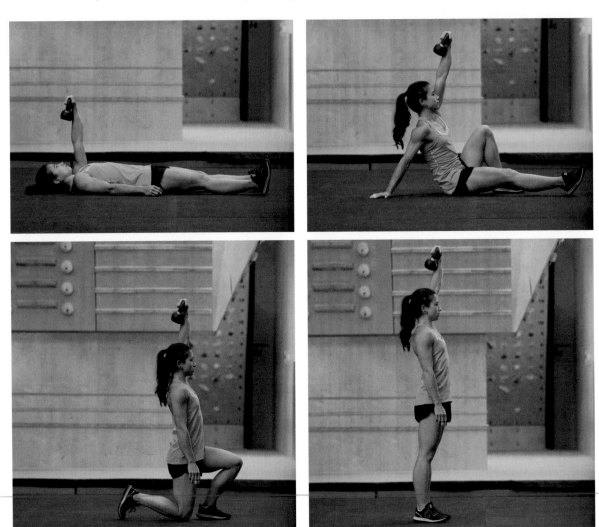

▶ *Turkish Getup*

leg back so that your right knee is on the floor under your hips. Keep a neutral spine with a lifted chest. In one smooth movement, straighten out the lower right leg so it's in line with your left leg and stand on your right knee. Then perform a split squat to stand upright with feet side by side. Go back down the exact opposite way you came up.

Straight-arm plank: Same as the forearm plank, but with arms straight and wrists directly underneath the shoulders.

Shoulder dislocate: Use something light, like a PVC pipe, or stretchy, like a therapy band. Flexible equipment allows for more wrist angles, but use whatever is comfortable—just not anything heavy. Grip wider than shoulder-width apart. The closer the grip, the more intense the stretch; start wide and gradually decrease the width with more practice. Lift the pipe or band over your head and back down behind you until it reaches hip height. Return and repeat for one minute.

ESSENTIAL YOGA POSES

With overdeveloped lats, shoulders pulled forward, strained necks, and tight hamstrings, it's amazing that climbers can function in daily life and on the wall. But there's a perfect solution to balance all that tightness out: yoga. It promotes balance, increases core strength, calms your mind, and teaches you how to be in your body. Of course you can go to pricey yoga classes at a studio, or check out the classes offered at your gym, but you can also practice on your own whenever you have time.

This is a great workout to do on a rest day, as it's very low intensity and gets the blood flowing, which aids in muscle recovery. The following poses focus on opening your chest and stretching your hamstrings, legs, and hips—all things that prevent injury.

The Workout

Try to "flow" all these poses together into one session, moving from each posture back to Mountain Pose, and then on to the next. Maintain steady breathing throughout your practice. Inhale as you establish the posture, and then breathe deeply and rhythmically as you hold the pose. Before you initiate any movement, relax and focus on your breath.

Start by standing, expanding your full back with a deep breath and lengthening the sides of your body. Always begin with and return to Mountain Pose. Hold each pose for thirty to sixty seconds. Do asymmetrical poses on each side. Don't strive for maximum extension, especially if you are new to yoga. Focus on standing up tall, without sticking your buttocks or chest out.

The Exercises

Mountain Pose

Body benefits: This is your basic yoga "ready" pose. It promotes stillness, relaxed strength, and "groundedness." Think of yourself as a mountain.

▶ Stand with heels slightly apart, big toes touching. Balance your weight evenly by lifting and spreading your toes and rocking your body over your feet.

▶ Lift your kneecaps, strengthen the inner arches of your feet, turn the upper thighs slightly inward, and draw your pubic bone and tailbone toward each other.

▶ Lift your upper body without sticking your ribs out, stretch your shoulder blades back, and drop your shoulders.

▶ Drop and straighten your arms, opening your palms in front of you.

▶ Grow tall through the crown of your head, chin parallel to the floor.

▶ Allow your tongue to be flat on the floor of your mouth.

▶ "Soften" your eyes: They should be open but slightly unfocused, so your gaze is relaxed.

Eagle Pose

Body benefits: Stretches latissimus dorsi, trapezius, and deltoid muscles.

Caution: People with knee pain should simply stand or cross one ankle over the other, leaving both feet touching the ground.

▶ With knees slightly bent, lift your left foot and balance on your right.

▶ Reach up with your arms and sink into your hips to create a sense of the spine lengthening and straightening.

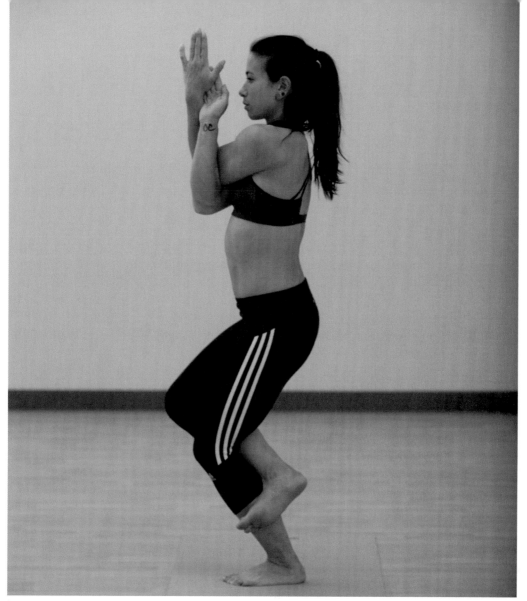

▶ *Eagle Pose*

    ▶ Cross your right thigh over the left, right toes pointed to the floor. Then, try to wrap the top of your right foot around the lower left calf. Hips face forward.

    ▶ Cross your forearms, placing your left above right, and bend the elbows. Press the inside of your right hand against the lower part of the palm of your left hand.

    ▶ Raise the arms and bend at the elbows so that the upper arms are parallel to the ground, fingers stretched upward.

Warrior Pose I

Body benefits: Strengthens and stretches your quadriceps, hamstrings, and hip flexors.

Caution: Those with lower-back disc issues should narrow the stance.

▶ Reach your left leg back and bend your right knee directly over your right ankle.

▶ Place your left foot flat at a 45-degree angle. Make sure your right ankle and foot are at a 90-degree angle (pointing forward), and that your right heel is aligned with your left heel. (People with ankle problems may lift the heel and balance on the toes.)

▶ Draw your right, outer hip back, and align your right thigh parallel to the ground.

▶ Lift your torso and arch your upper back slightly, while raising arms overhead.

▶ Point fingers up with palms facing together. Lift your rib cage away from the pelvis.

▶ Look forward, head in a neutral position.

▶ Repeat on the other side, with your left leg forward and right leg back.

Downward-Facing Dog Pose (aka Down Dog)

Body benefits: Strengthens and stretches shoulder muscles, strengthens latissimus dorsi, and stretches hamstrings, calf muscles, and Achilles tendon. Helps prevent rotator cuff injuries.

Caution: People with shoulder problems shouldn't do this posture without expert supervision.

▶ Drop to your hands and knees with your knees directly below your hips.

▶ Spread your hands wide and slightly in front of your shoulders, with index fingers slightly turned out.

▶ Lift your buttocks and slowly straighten your legs, without locking your knees.

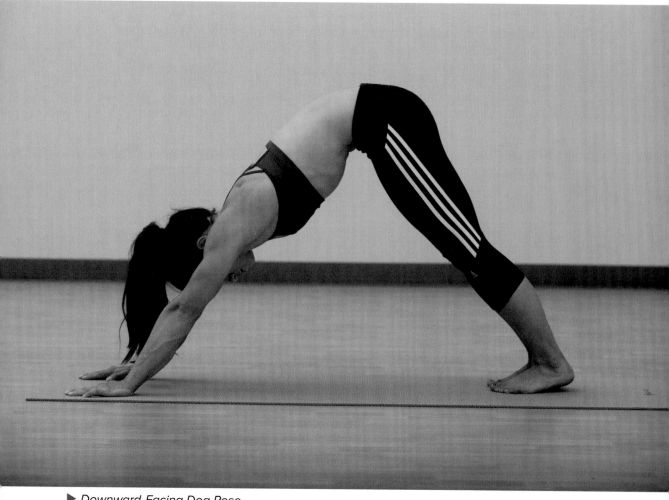

▶ *Downward-Facing Dog Pose*

▶ Stretch your heels down. It's OK if your heels don't touch the floor and if your legs remain slightly bent.

▶ Press the base of the index fingers firmly into the floor, and lift your inner arms.

▶ Pull your shoulder blades away from your ears, broadening the collarbone.

▶ Do not allow your head to hang; keep it between your upper arms.

Seated Twist

Body benefits: Strengthens and stretches the back. Strengthens shoulder muscles. Opens shoulders by stretching pectoral muscles.

▶ Sit evenly on your sit bones and straighten your back. If your lower back is sagging, prop yourself up on a folded blanket.

▶ Extend your legs in front of you without locking your knees.

▶ Bend your right knee, and place your right foot at on the ground outside of your left knee.

▶ Bend your left leg, with your ankle close to the right hip.

▶ Lift your right arm and stretch the side of your body, while twisting your torso to the right. Place your right hand or fingers on the ground behind you.

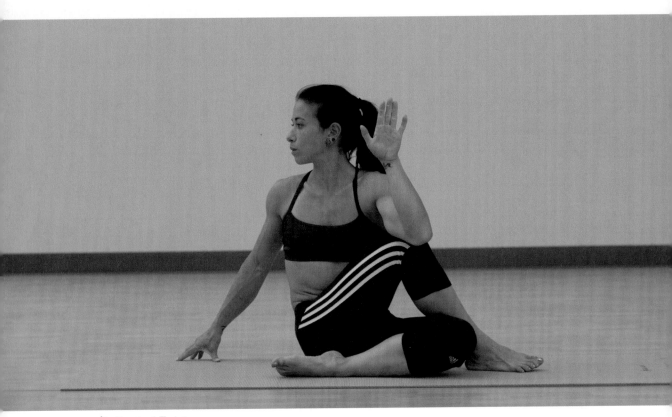

▶ *Seated Twist*

- Lift your left arm and place the outside of your left elbow on the outside of your right knee to help maintain the twist. However, be sure to move from the base of your spine as you twist. Do not force the twist with the strength of your arms.

- Look over your right shoulder.

- Repeat on other side.

Bridge Pose
Body benefits: Strengthens spine and gluteus maximus. Stretches and opens muscles in the chest, neck, and spine, which climbers compress and contract through constant pulling. Stretches psoas muscles, which connect the lower spine to the pelvis.

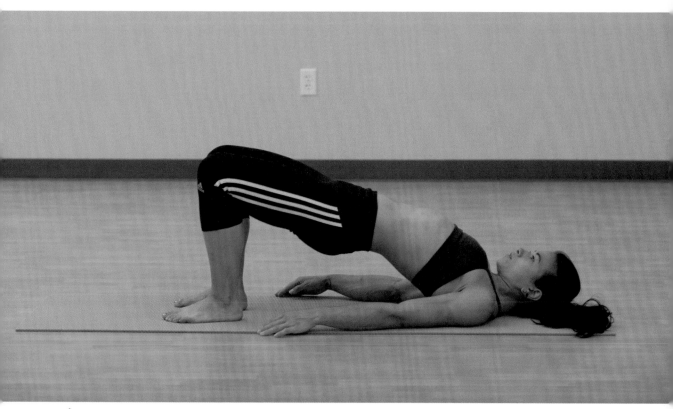

▶ *Bridge Pose*

Caution: If you have a neck injury, do not do this pose without expert supervision.

► Lie at on your back, arms by your sides.

► Bend your knees and bring your heels close to your buttocks.

► Lift your chest and raise your hips, keeping your thighs parallel to each other. Don't clench your buttocks.

► Press your feet into the ground, and draw your knees forward over your ankles as you lift your pelvis and lengthen your tailbone.

► Clasp your hands together under your back and stay high on your shoulders.

► Lift your chest, chin away from the sternum, and push your head into the floor.

► Tuck your tailbone while broadening your back and shoulder blades. Firm your entire body.

► Roll the spine slowly down to release from the pose.

Wide-Legged Standing Forward Bend
Body benefits: Loosens hamstrings, opens shoulders, and finds midline for greater stability. Lengthens the spine.

► Stand sideways on your mat with your feet wide apart.

► Turn your thighs and big toes in slightly.

► Interlock your fingers at your sacrum. Keep some space between your wrists.

► Press evenly into the four corners of your feet, fold forward at your hips, and take your arms overhead, sliding them toward the floor.

► Experiment with turning your palms toward your back (which will open your superficial shoulder muscles and fascia) or turning them out and externally rotating your shoulders.

► Stay for five breaths. Come up to standing and bring your feet together.

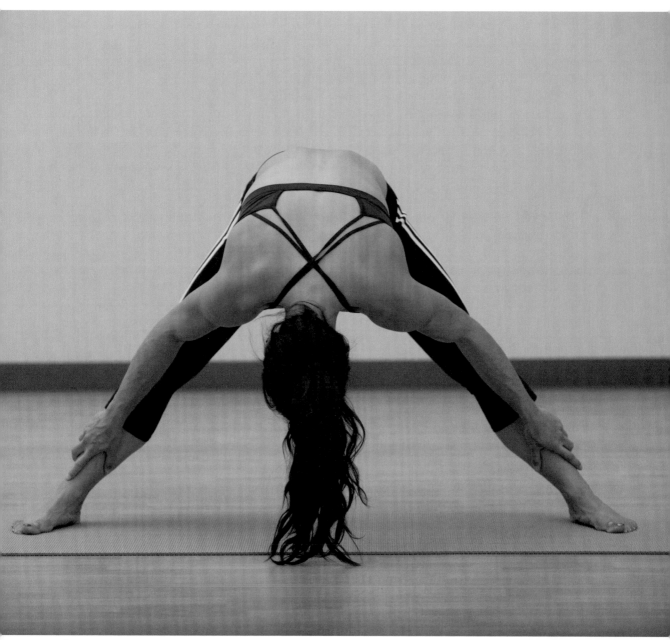

▶ *Wide-Legged Standing Forward*

One-Legged King Pigeon Pose

Body benefits: Opens outer hips and thighs. Stretches the inner groin, a tight spot for climbers. Softens the hip flexors of the back leg and will give you space to reach those high footholds.

▶ From Down Dog, lift your right leg into the air.

▶ Bend that leg and bring the knee toward your right wrist, setting the side of your lower leg on the ground and forming an angle with your right shin and thigh bone.

▶ Inch your hips back by turning your left toes under and picking up your hips and setting them down evenly.

▶ Come down onto your elbows or forehead, and relax into a forward fold over your right shin.

▶ Keep some energy pulling inward as you release the big muscles of your right hip.

▶ Stay for at least one minute and up to five minutes.

▶ Release, and assume the pose on the other side.

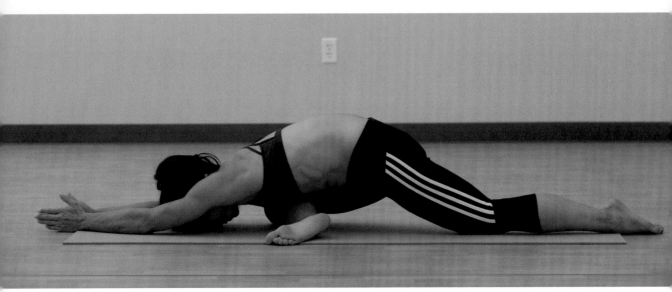

▶ *One-Legged King Pigeon Pose*

Tree Pose

Body benefits: Helps you finds your center. Improves mental focus and balance. Opens the hips.

▶ From standing, shift your body weight onto your left leg and lift your right leg off the floor.

▶ Place the sole of your right foot as high on the inner left thigh as you can (above or below the knee, but never on your knee).

▶ Open the right hip.

▶ Press the right foot into the left thigh.

▶ Find your midline and press your standing leg into the ground; feel your spine grow long out of this rootedness.

▶ Hold for five deep breaths.

▶ Release, and repeat on the other side.

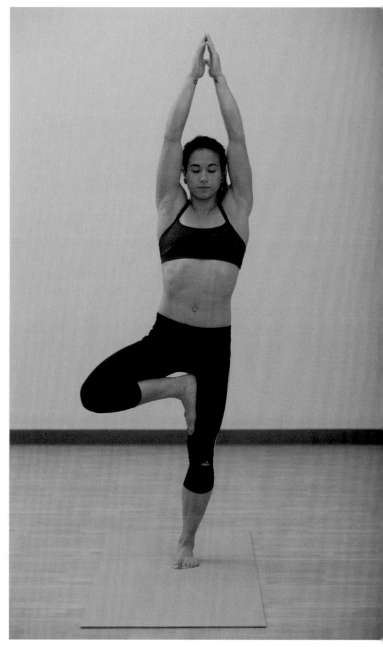

▶ *Tree Pose*

Side Plank Pose

Body benefits: Tones arms, shoulders, and core.

▶ From Down Dog, slide your right hand a few inches to the right, toward your midline.

▶ Turn onto the outside edge of your right foot, and stack your ankles on top of each other.

▶ Roll your hips open to the left, and without sagging, open your left arm toward the sky.

▶ Imagine a magnetic pull connecting the inner lines of your legs; this supports your spine. To wake up your external obliques and serratus muscles, imagine wrapping the right side of your rib cage toward your left front hip bone.

▶ Keep your shoulder blades and collarbones wide. Puff up the space in between your shoulder blades.

▶ Stay for five breaths, then transfer your weight through Plank Pose, Down Dog, and to the other side.

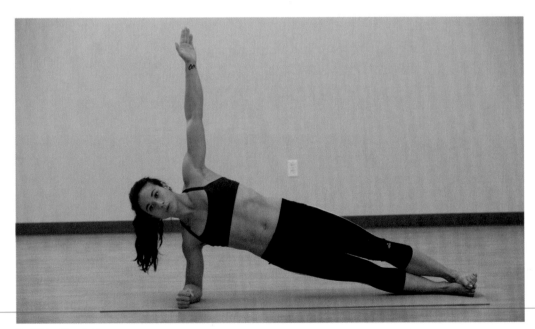

▶ *Side Plank Pose*

LONG-TERM PROGRAM: SHOULDER AND HIP STRENGTHENING

All athletic movement starts with the hips and core; strong hips equal a strong athlete. Shoulders are the most sophisticated joints in the body; they have a wide range of motion and need to be strong at any and all weird angles for the extreme movements required in climbing. The key is training hard and smart—with a specific plan—so you can see real gains instead of just fatigue.

This plan focuses on the hips and shoulders, and should be done any time you need to take a break from climbing. It's perfect for people who have nagging finger injuries but can still lift weights safely. You will go hard for three weeks, and pull it back during the fourth week. This means going through the same motions, but concentrating on muscle endurance for all exercises.

THE WORKOUT

The exercises for strength versus endurance are the same, but the sets, reps, and weight differ. On each training day, do one strength exercise, and then fill in the rest of the session with three muscular endurance exercises for the opposite part of the body (pick from the list of recommended exercises or add your own). For example, choose one upper body exercise and do that as your strength movement, and then perform three lower body endurance exercises that allow your upper body to recover. Add two days a week of cardio conditioning as well; one day should be challenging but short, and one should be long and slow. Sprints, jogging, rowing, cycling, and swimming are good choices for both, as you can change the intensity based on your goal. Weight train four days a week; two of those days should include cardio conditioning. Rest one full day per week, and on the other two days you can climb, rest, or do some combination of both.

▶ Strength: Three sets of one to five reps at heavy load (85 percent of max for all reps) for each exercise; rest at least three minutes between sets; add 2.5 to 5 pounds each week.

▶ Endurance: Three sets of twelve (or more) reps for each exercise (about 50 to 65 percent of max); rest thirty seconds to three minutes between sets; each rep should be fluid (two seconds up, two seconds down, with zero rest at the bottom and top); only add weight if you can complete each rep at this pace.

THE EXERCISES

▶ Upper body: Standing press, dips, pull-ups, bent-over rows, closed-grip pull-ups, push press, bench press, offset pull-ups, one-arm press

▶ Lower body: Deadlifts, one-leg deadlifts, back squats, Cossack squats, front squats, weighted lunges, weighted step-ups, kettlebell swings, Bulgarian split squats (see Bulgarian Lunges, page 155)

Hip and Shoulder Strengthening Tips

▶ Have a coach at your local climbing gym teach you proper form while training, and help you safely figure out your max for each lift.

▶ Warm up and cool down with ten minutes of active stretching and/or a few minutes of jogging.

▶ A training partner will help keep you accountable and motivated.

▶ Take at least one full rest day a week.

▶ Start with a weight that's about 85 percent of your max for strength, so you can make great gains but still recover.

▶ The more muscles used in each movement, the better, because climbing requires coordinated efforts from multiple body parts for every move (i.e., avoid exercises that isolate specific muscles, like bicep curls).

▶ Most exercises can be done unilaterally (using one side of the body at a time), which more closely mimics actual climbing.

SAMPLE WORKOUT WEEK

Repeat for three weeks; the fourth week is the same movements, but all endurance.

MONDAY

Standing press (upper body strength); deadlift, kettlebell swings, weighted step-ups (lower body endurance)

TUESDAY

Rest or go climbing

WEDNESDAY

Back squats (lower body strength); standing press, dips, push press (upper body endurance)

THURSDAY

Rest or go climbing

FRIDAY

Bench press (upper body strength); one-leg deadlifts, Cossack squats, weighted lunges (lower-body endurance)

SATURDAY

Rest or go climbing

SUNDAY

Deadlifts (lower body strength); standing press, bent-over rows, closed-grip pull-ups (upper body endurance)

This 4-week Shoulder and Hip Strengthening plan will help you do just that: get stronger hips and shoulders, both areas that climbers tend to ignore for strength training. If you've been focusing on climbing-specific training for a while, this is a great way to switch things up but maintain a workout regimen in the gym. This can also be a good workout if you're dealing with finger injuries. Just take the rest days instead of climbing.

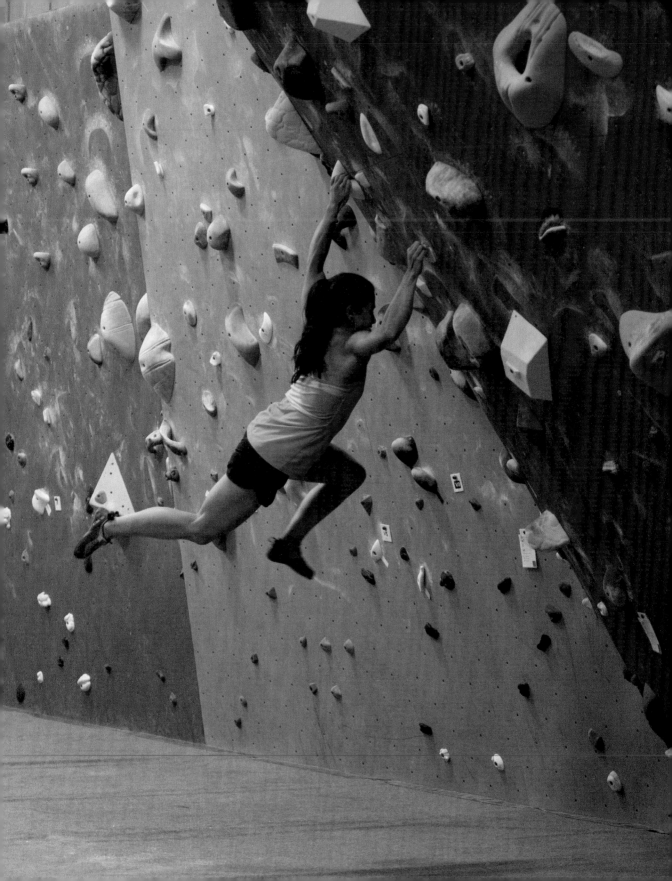

Chapter 6

CLIMB A GRADE HARDER

ANY TIME YOU CLIMB AT THE GYM, you're improving your overall fitness by burning calories, working your muscles, and just generally being active. But the key to any fitness program, climbing or otherwise, is consistency. Any mishmash of strength, cardio, climbing, and weight training will make you stronger—as long as you're consistent. This chapter offers just that by giving you a list of workouts and exercises to do every day, even if it's just a "take a rest day" (aka "doing nothing"). It contains a nine-week course, designed by renowned climbing coach Justen Sjong, to help you improve your climbing by a full grade. If you now climb 5.9 to 5.11, or V0 to V3, and follow this course down to the letter, you will climb a full grade harder after nine weeks. You can focus on bouldering or roped climbing, toprope or lead; this program works for all of it.

This program also focuses on two main skills in climbing: your eyes and your breath. When your eyes and your breath are in sync, you can tap into a new level of body awareness and climbing skill. You will reinforce this through fitness training, so that where you focus your eyes and breath becomes instinctual. This program also focuses on your specific climbing goals, which are important to keep in mind every day you train. Take time at the start of the program to write down your goals, so that each day you go into the gym you have the same goal and mission.

Many of the workouts and exercises are repeated throughout the longer program. The first time an exercise appears, there is a detailed explanation of how to do it, what to focus on, and some extra tips. Each following appearance just has the name of the exercise and a page number. As you work through the program, you might need a reminder on how to perform the movements. Use the page numbers to refer back to the original explanation of the exercise.

A basic breakdown of the nine weeks:

▶ Week 1: Figuring out your baseline

▶ Week 2: Improving baseline fitness

▶ Week 3: Exploring Contrast

▶ Week 4: Improving finger strength

▶ Week 5: Rest and recover

▶ Week 6: Increasing intensity

▶ Week 7: Trying your hardest

▶ Week 8: Matching mental game with performance

▶ Week 9: Reaching peak performance

The daily structure is laid out below, but life obligations can get in the way, partners can flake, and every climber's schedule is a little different. It's totally fine to swap days just as long as you complete each week's work before moving on to the next, and you don't climb on back-to-back days. While the program is built on a Monday-to-Sunday schedule, you can adapt to what works best for your life. If you're consistent week in and week out, you will get physically stronger.

General Schedule

We started the schedule on a Monday, but feel free to adapt to whatever start day works best for you.

▶ **Monday:** Rest

▶ **Tuesday:** Roped climbing*

▶ **Wednesday:** Fitness

▶ **Thursday:** Bouldering

▶ **Friday:** Rest

▶ **Weekend:** Climb for fun, hang out with your friends and family, enjoy your weekend however you want!

*Within the program, there will be alternate activities on Tuesdays for those who wish to focus solely on bouldering.

WARM-UP

Warming up is something that you will do every day you climb. Many people dread warming up, but this is the part when you become awesome. Do not rush this process—take the time to find your confidence, your strut. Make purposeful eye contact with the holds, and develop the ideal breath.

The warm-up process starts off super easy. Do a problem or route, come down, and then think about how it went. Did it feel perfect, or were there changes you would have made? Climb the exact same route again. Part of the warm-up should be about warming up the "Grr"—the try-hard. We don't go from zero to sixty naturally. We have to warm up that engine. Take the time and learn to rev as you warm up.

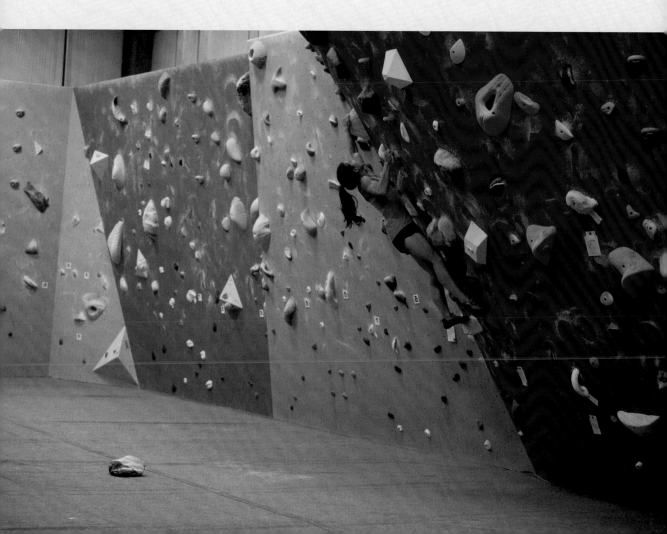

WARM-UP STEPS

1. Start off easy. "Easy" and "hard" are relative terms. Even the strongest climbers like to traverse using any foot, wandering on large holds. The initial goal is to see how you're feeling and moving today.

2. Transition onto designated/graded climbs, but don't feel obligated to finish them or stay on the taped holds.

3. Get all your systems in sync: the eyes, breath, coordination, and anything that helps you feel confident on the wall. Slowly increase difficulty until you have to try. If you're feeling good, start on harder problems; if you're feeling bad, drop down to relocate your confidence. You determine the pace and duration. Some can get the job done in twenty minutes, while others need an hour.

4. Rest up. Rest is something that should happen in three- to ten-minute blocks; make sure to take your shoes off so you mentally transition into rest mode.

5. Record your climbs in a small notebook so you can reflect back on your method: what works, what doesn't.

WEEK 1: FIGURING OUT YOUR BASELINE

This week is all about finding your base level of fitness: Where are you in the climbing world? To achieve your goal, you'll need to know exactly where you're starting from. That means establishing your top four routes and your top six boulder problems, meaning the hardest four or six climbs you can complete in one session.

When you're warming up, the goal is to become awesome. If you want to send your top climbs, you need to feel good, you need to feel confident. Take the time to identify what your strength is and what your confidence looks like. Do this before you touch the first hold. Pause a minute, take a few deep breaths, and shift your mindset to being strong and confident. Then, when you're on the climb, how you chalk up, how you move, how you pause become really important. Enjoy doing nothing for a second; enjoy looking at that next hold that you're going crush. You have to look at it and want it—you're going to grab it and bear down on it. Learn to connect with your eyes and your breath.

For the sake of this example, we started the programs in this chapter on a Monday. If you start on another day, adjust accordingly. Refer to this handy chart for a quick at-a-glance view of the week, with daily descriptions to follow. This schedule starts with a rest day; that's assuming you had an active weekend. If you didn't, consider starting Monday with Tuesday's workout, etc.

WEEK 1	
Monday	Rest day
Tuesday	Find Your Baseline
	• Warm-up
	• Top 4 Routes / Top 6 Problems
Wednesday	Fitness day
	• Cardio
	• Band routine
	• Wrist routine
Thursday	Climbing day
	• Warm-up
	• Bouldering: Top 6 Problems
Friday	Rest day
Weekend	Climb for Fun Day
	• Warm-up

Monday

Monday is a rest day—this assumes you are climbing one day each weekend.

Tuesday

Find your average climbing grade (aka your baseline).

▶ Warm-up

▶ Top 4 Routes*

If you are focused on bouldering, you'll do Top 6 Problems instead.

Top 4 Routes / Top 6 Problems

This is an average of the four hardest grades you can climb in one session, which establishes your climbing baseline. Do this on toprope or lead, whichever you'd like to focus on for the program. It is important that you complete all four. They won't all be your best climbs ever, but you should try to do the best job possible. If you fall, repeat that route to try to get that send; it's important that you get those sends. Your top four climbs will give you an average that will give you a sense of where you are. If you're focused on bouldering, do your Top 6 Problems instead. Same idea though: average the difficulty of the six hardest problems you can complete.

Wednesday

Day three is a fitness day. The program:

▶ Cardio (running, stationary bike, rowing machine—your choice)

▶ Band routine (three exercises)

▶ Wrist routine (four exercises)

Cardio

It's part of the fitness day warm-up. Do twenty to thirty minutes of cardio on the torture device of your choosing: stationary bike, treadmill, elliptical, or rowing machine. You could even go for a short hike. Start off with low intensity and build up to high intensity. It's about gaining heart fitness.

Band Routine

These three exercises—the internal, external, and elevated rotations—are designed to strengthen your shoulders, which can be a problem area for climbers if they don't do focused shoulder work. Do fifteen reps for two to three sets each, with no rest between exercises but a one-minute rest between sets. Start with an easy band and slowly work up over the course of the program. You're aiming for a nice even burn in your shoulders after the last set. If your band is too heavy, you're targeting the wrong muscles.

Band exercises:

▶ Internal rotations: Elbow stays tucked into your trunk; pull the band across your body. Then you're going to transition straight into the external.

▶ External rotations: Using the same arm, turn your body around so you're facing the other way. Elbow stays tucked; pull the band out away from your body.

▶ Elevated rotations: You may or may not use a band for these. Elbows are straight out, bent at 90 degrees, and your palms face the floor. Rotate at the shoulders to lift your hands so the fingers point up and palms face forward, then lower them again to face the floor.

Wrist Routine

When hangboarding, which you'll be getting to in subsequent weeks, the wrist is a weak point. These four exercises—the wrist rotation, curl, extension, and roller—are designed to keep your wrists strong and happy. Do two to four sets, fifteen reps each. Pick a weight that will give you an even burn after the last set.

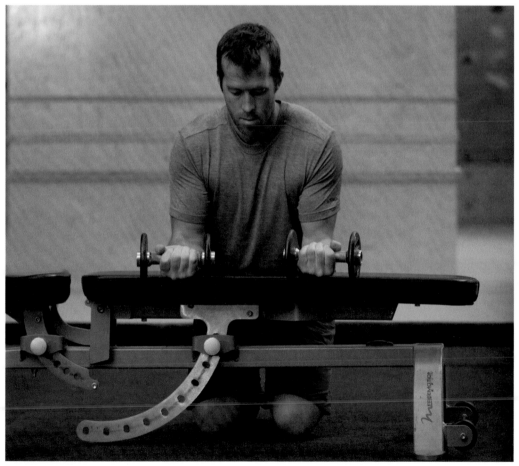

▶ *Wrist Curls*

- ▶ Wrist rotation: Start with wrist rotation. Hold a dumbbell in the middle and slowly spin it left, then right, keeping your forearm supported by a bench. Go straight into wrist curls.

- ▶ Wrist curls: Drop the dumbbell all the way down (as far as it will go based on the flexibility of your wrist), and then spin it back up. You might need a lighter weight for wrist extension.

- ▶ Wrist extension: Lift the back side of your wrist up and drop it back down in a controlled fashion.

- ▶ Wrist roller: Use the wrist-roller device. Hold it straight in front of you. With elbows slightly bent, spin the weight up to the PVC pipe. Hold it there for a split second, then reverse it back down. Bring it back up again, etc.

Thursday

Back to climbing. Today's program:

- ▶ Warm-up (page 198)

- ▶ Bouldering: Top 6 Problems

Bouldering: Top 6 Problems

Whether you're focused on roped climbing or bouldering, you'll average the difficulty of the six hardest problems you can complete. If you're focusing on roped climbing, the power you develop while bouldering translates to completing hard moves on longer routes. If you already did the Top 6 Problems on Tuesday, try to do them again, focusing on the eyes, breath, and your confidence even more than the first time. Don't necessarily try to raise your baseline, but try to see and feel the difference between today's session and the Tuesday session.

Friday

Friday is a rest day. Enjoy resting up after three days of hard work, and start figuring out your weekend climbing plan and lining up a partner. Enjoy yourself. You deserve it.

Weekend

Do whatever you want, but plan to climb on either Saturday or Sunday just for fun. Of course, don't forget to warm up. However, if you're feeling mentally or physically fatigued, take a break from climbing to explore another active outdoor pursuit, like skiing, hiking, or biking.

WEEK 2: IMPROVING BASELINE FITNESS

This week, you'll build on your baseline fitness while also working on your ground game and getting into the zone.

Your ground game plays out immediately after a climb, when you come back down and recall what just happened. Don't just visualize with your eyes and picture the climb from above. Try to feel what you just did. Was it good? Was it bad? Where did you go astray? What was the source of the problem? Where were you awesome? If you did great, celebrate that. You need to focus on three things during the reflection process: what happened; what you need; how you get it.

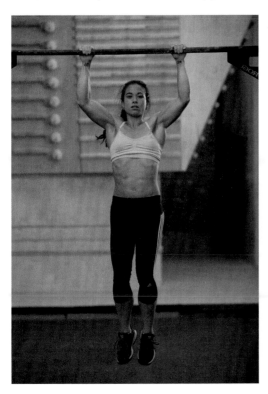 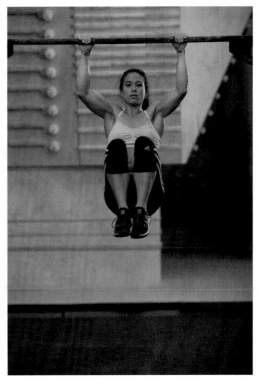

WEEK 2	
Monday	Rest day
Tuesday	Work on Your Ground Game
	• Warm-up
	• Route doubles or boulder repeaters
	• Three block exercises
	• Shoulder IYTs
Wednesday	Fitness day
Thursday	Climbing day
	• Warm-up
	• Bouldering hard/easy
	• Three block exercises
	• Wrist routine
Friday	Rest day
Weekend	Climb for Fun Day
	• Warm-up

Monday

Rest day.

Tuesday

Work on your ground game. Get in the zone and build on your baseline. The program:

▶ Warm-up

▶ Route doubles or boulder repeaters (choose the latter if you have a bouldering-only focus)

• Choose routes at or near your onsight level

• Do two climbs

• Take eight- to fifteen-minute rests between sets

• 2–5 sets

- ▶ These three exercises* are done in a block, which makes them a single set.

  - Negative pull-ups (60 seconds); rest 30 seconds

  - Knee tucks (60 seconds); rest 30 seconds

  - Drop-roll-jumps (60 seconds)

  - Rest three minutes and repeat for 2–4 sets

The goal is not to complete the full minute. The goal is to stay aware and correct course when your form or quality drops. Being tired is OK, but lazy behavior is not OK.

- ▶ Shoulder IYTs

  - 0–5 pounds

  - Fifteen reps

  - Three-minute rests between sets

  - 2–4 sets

Route Doubles/Bouldering Repeaters

Climb one great problem or route (toprope or lead), and after you're done, reflect briefly on what went well and what didn't. Then climb it again right away, but don't rush. Go when you're ready (not fully rested), and try to climb it better.

Negative Pull-Ups

With hands shoulder-width apart, pull up on a bar like normal, then aim for a three- to five-count on the lower. When your arms are fully extended, take a breath. Repeat. Especially in the beginning, you will not be able to complete a full minute. Form is everything, so push yourself and try hard, but when your form suffers, stop.

Knee Tucks

Hang on a pull-up bar with hands shoulder-width apart and elbows slightly bent, which will help engage your core. Tuck your knees up into your waist and back down. Keep your toes pointed. Repeat this motion, pausing when you need to.

Drop-Roll-Jumps

These build core strength and explosive leg energy. Form matters for this athletic movement. Start standing, then drop down to the ground on a soft surface. Roll back so your feet go over your head, then kip forward. Tuck your heels back toward your

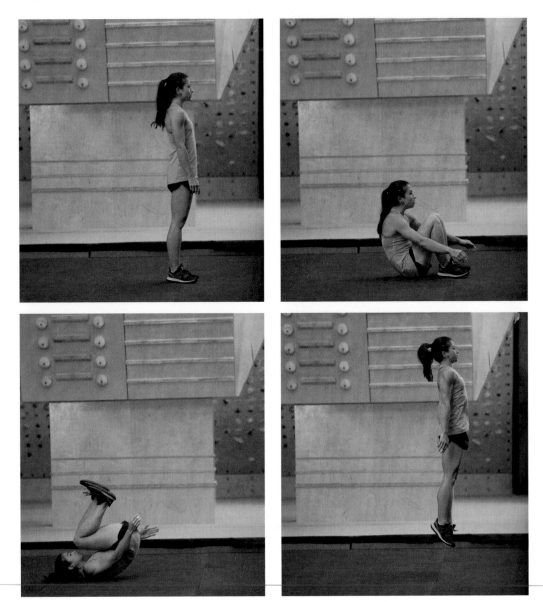

▶ Drop-roll-jump sequence.

butt, then stand up quickly and go straight into a jump. Right when you come back down, flow right back into the Drop-Roll-Jump. Things to look out for: When you go back into the roll and you roll forward, your heels need to be toward your hips. If they're too far in front of you, you're going to have to use your hands to push yourself back up and you're going to spring-load backward. Make sure your heels are close to you. Jump. When you jump, point your toes, and move your hands above your head.

Shoulder IYTs

These are about strengthening your upper, inner back. Use a 45-degree bench, with your belly on the bench, and focus on squeezing your inner back with all of these movements. Choose a light weight to get a nice, even burn throughout your body, not lifting for strength. Transition directly from Is to Ys to Ts, doing five of each. Face your thumbs straight up for the Is; lift straight up above your head. Transition straight into the Ys, thumbs going straight out. For the Ts, flip your thumbs so they're internal, pull them back, and squeeze your inner back.

Wednesday

Fitness day. The program:

▶ Cardio (20 minutes)

- These six exercises* are done in a block, which makes it a single set.

- Push-ups (60 seconds); rest 30 seconds

- Scissors (60 seconds); rest 30 seconds

- Right-side plank (60 seconds); rest 30 seconds

- Left-side plank (60 seconds); rest 30 seconds

- Leg lift (60 seconds); rest 30 seconds

- Air squats (60 seconds)

- Rest three minutes and repeat for 2–4 sets

The goal is not to complete the full minute for each exercise. The goal is to stay aware and correct course when your form or quality drops. Being tired is OK, but lazy behavior is not OK.

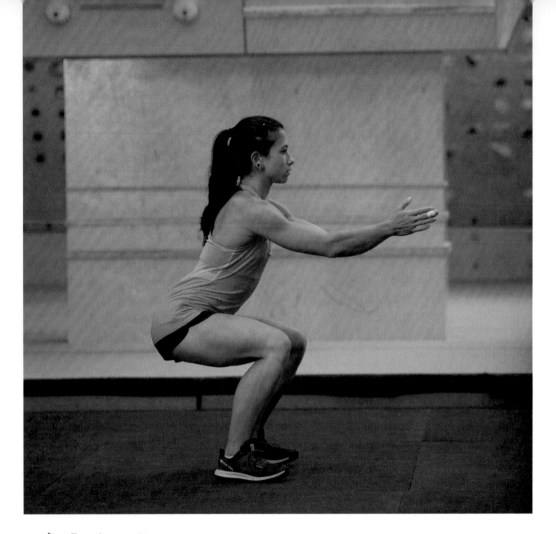

▶ Band exercises

- Easy band

- Three exercises, no rest between exercises

- Fifteen reps each

- Three-minute rest between sets

- 2–4 sets

Push-Ups

Form really matters. The key part about push-ups is to have your palms underneath your shoulders, with elbows 45 degrees from your trunk. Complete an even push-up, then an even push-down. Be very aware of where your lower back and your hips are. You want a nice, solid, flat back; no sagging. Do push-ups on a hard surface, not a soft surface like a climbing floor, which is terrible for your wrists. Everyone gets tired at some point. Have the discipline to bump down to your knees when needed. Be very aware of where your lower back is, even on your knees. Do these for a full minute, pausing when you need to pause. When your form starts to go downhill, bump down to your knees or even stop. Compose yourself, drop your gaze, feel your breath, and then begin again.

Scissors

Do this core workout in a controlled fashion with toes pointed. With your hands behind your lower back, arch your neck forward, with your toes pointed out in front of you. Cross your feet back and forth. When you start flopping around, stop. Take a breath. Your core is engaged the whole time and your feet need to stay a certain distance—ideally about 18 inches—above the ground.

Side Planks

This is another great core exercise. Lie on your side, propping your forearm underneath your shoulder. Your feet are stacked on top of each other, hips in a straight line with your shoulders and legs. When you get fatigued, it is very natural for your hips to sag too low, and then for you to start overcompensating and arch the hips too high. Keep a nice even plane from your shoulders down to your toes.

Leg Lifts

Build on knee tucks by bringing your legs straight out in front of you. Place your hands shoulder-width apart on a pull-up bar, with a slight bend in the elbows. With toes pointed, bring your feet straight out in front of you and hold there for a millisecond. Drop your legs in a controlled, gentle swing, lift back up, and repeat.

Air Squats

With feet shoulder-width apart and weight on your heels (try to lift your toes), squat down like you would to sit in a chair. Spike back up with authority, and land in a standing position. Then squat back down to repeat the movement.

Thursday

Today is a bouldering and fitness day. Here is the program:

▶ Warm-up (page 198)

▶ Bouldering hard/easy

- Hard = around your project level. Easy = a grade that would be an early warm-up

- 2 boulders

- 4- to 10-minute rests between sets

- 2–7 sets

▶ These three exercises* are done in a block, which makes it a single set.

- Negative pull-ups (60 seconds); rest 30 seconds (page 205)

- Knee tucks (60 seconds); rest 30 seconds (page 205)

- Drop-roll-jumps (60 seconds) (page 206)

- Rest three minutes and repeat for 2–4 sets

The goal is not to complete the full minute. The goal is to stay aware and correct course when your form or quality drops. Being tired is OK, but lazy behavior is not OK.

▶ Wrist routine (page 201)

- Use light weight

- Four exercises, no rest between exercises

- Fifteen reps each

- Three-minute rests between sets

- 2–4 sets

Bouldering Hard/Easy

In this exercise, you are feeling the contrast between having a problem dialed and working hard. Choose two good problems, one hard and one easy. You should be able to finish the hard one, and the easy one should be very easy. You are feeling the contrast between high intensity and low intensity. From across the room, a friend should be able to identify which one was hard and which one was easy for you. Climb a hard one, then an easy one. Rest. Repeat hard then easy for two to seven sets, picking new problems for each set.

Friday
This is a rest day.

Weekend
Climb for fun at least one day, two if you'd like, or do another moderate activity for one day, such as a hike or a bike ride.

WEEK 3: EXPLORING CONTRAST

Build upon on Week 2 by exploring contrast: hard/easy, low intensity / high intensity, good/bad. By going through the same routine as Week 2, you'll get an opportunity to focus on this. Your eyes and your breath build this performance. The way you look at things determines the level of intensity. If you look at something with low intensity, your eyes should be soft, your eyebrows and eyelids relaxed. When our eyes are soft, we see the big picture. When you go up in intensity, your eyes and your brow become stern, and you become very singular. Learn to fluctuate between soft and big picture, and hard and singular. Blend in the idea of your breath helping you rev your engine, shifting through the gears. There's low intensity, your baseline, aka first gear. Then there are three more gears. Gear two is about power-endurance. Revving the engine, feeling the intensity. Then you have third gear, where you might make try-hard sounds because your output is near max

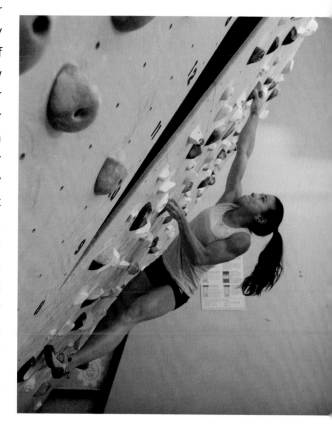

level. Fourth gear is holding your breath, where you're in control to the point of not breathing. All of these gears are important: You need to learn how to rev, how to drive these gears, and when to be in each gear.

WEEK 3	
Monday	Rest day
Tuesday	Feel the Contrast
	• Warm-up
	• Route doubles or boulder repeaters
	• Three block exercises
	• IYTs
Wednesday	Fitness day
Thursday	Feel the Contrast
	• Warm-up
	• Bouldering hard/easy
	• Three block exercises
	• Wrist routine
Friday	Rest day
Weekend	Climb for Fun Day
	• Warm-up

Monday
Monday each week is a rest day—this assumes you are climbing one day each weekend.

Tuesday
Feel the contrast. The program:

▶ Warm-up (page 198)

▶ Route doubles or boulder repeaters (choose the latter if you have a bouldering-only focus) (page 205)

- Choose routes at or near your onsight level

- Do two climbs

- Take eight- to fifteen-minute rests between sets

- 2–5 sets

- ▶ These three exercises* are done in a block, which makes them a single set.

  - • Negative pull-ups (60 seconds); rest 30 seconds

  - • Supermans (60 seconds); rest 30 seconds

  - • Drop-roll-jumps (60 seconds)

  - • Rest three minutes and repeat for 2–4 sets

*The goal is not to complete the full minute. The goal is to stay aware and correct course when your form or quality drops. Being tired is OK, but lazy behavior is not OK.

- ▶ IYTs (page 206)

  - • 0–5 pounds

  - • Fifteen reps

  - • Three-minute rests between sets

  - • 2–4 sets

Supermans

To strengthen your lower back, lie on your belly and extend your hands out in front of you, feet extended behind. Arch and lift your hands and feet at the same time.

Wednesday

Fitness day. The program:

- ▶ Cardio: By now, you should aim to do 30 minutes of cardio on fitness days.

- ▶ These six exercises are done in a block, which makes them a single set.

  - • Push-ups (60 seconds); rest 30 seconds

  - • Leg lifts (60 seconds); rest 30 seconds

  - • Right-side plank (60 seconds); rest 30 seconds

  - • Left-side plank (60 seconds); rest 30 seconds

- V-ups (60 seconds); rest 30 seconds

- Air squats (60 seconds)

- Rest for three minutes, and repeat for 2–4 sets

The goal is not to complete the full minute. The goal is to stay aware and correct course when your form or quality drops. Being tired is OK, but lazy behavior is not OK.

▶ Band exercises

- Easy band

- Three exercises, no rest between exercises

- Fifteen reps each

- Three-minute rests between sets

- 2–4 sets

V-ups

This is a powerful core workout. These are difficult. Lie down on your back with your arms overhead. Spike your hands and feet up over your belly at the same time.

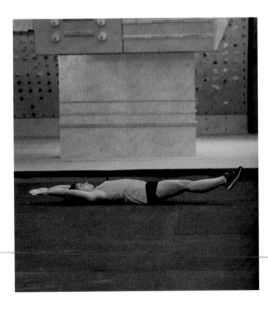
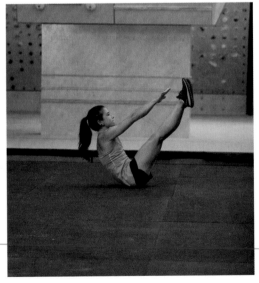

Then relax both back down, but don't allow your hands to touch the ground during a true V-up. Repeat, resting when needed. You might have to do an easier version: Instead of bringing your toes all the way up, bring your knees in toward your body.

Thursday

Keep feeling the contrast. The program:

- ▶ Warm-up (page 198)

- ▶ Bouldering hard/easy (page 210)

    - Hard = around your project level; easy = a grade considered an early warm-up

    - Two boulders

    - 4- to 10-minute rests between sets

    - 2–7 sets

- ▶ These three exercises* are done in a block, which makes a single set.

    - Jumping pull-ups (60 seconds); rest 30 seconds

    - Supermans (60 seconds); rest 30 seconds

    - Drop-roll jumps (60 seconds)

    - Rest three minutes and repeat for 2–4 sets

The goal is not to complete the full minute. The goal is to stay aware and correct course when your form or quality drops. Being tired is OK, but lazy behavior is not OK.

- ▶ Wrist routine (page 201)

    - Light weight

    - Four exercises; no rest between exercises

    - Fifteen reps each

    - Three-minute rests between sets

    - 2–4 sets

Jumping Pull-ups

Jumping pull-ups are an excellent drill for building strength because you suffer a lot. Place your hands shoulder-width apart on a pull-up bar. You will need a box to stand on. Adjust the box so you're grabbing the pull-up bar with a slight bend in your arms. This allows you to drop down and drive through your entire body when you jump. Pull up so you're hitting the bar to your chest. When you come down, lower in a controlled fashion. Don't lower so slowly that you're doing a negative pull-up, but don't smack the box when you land. Aim for a soft descent. This exercise uses your entire body; as your upper body gets tired, you're still using your lower body.

Friday

Rest day.

Weekend

Climb for fun at least one day, two if you'd like, or do another moderate activity for one day, such as a hike or a bike ride.

WEEK 4: IMPROVING FINGER STRENGTH

This week builds finger strength through a hangboard routine and bouldering. Bouldering is mainly projecting, which is a safe and athletic way to gain finger strength. Any time you focus on finger strength, don't overdo it. Your fingers and tendons are fragile. They function like muscles as we strengthen them—we tear them down and rebuild them—but with muscles, there's a lot more blood flow, so recovery is quicker. Take it slow.

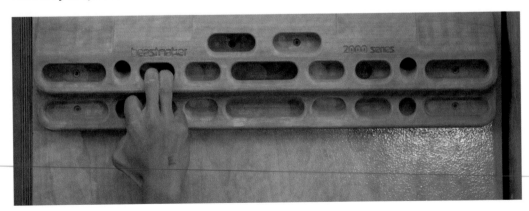

A second focus this week is on the relationship between your elbow and your breath. When your elbow is straight, you will find a nice calm breath. As soon as that elbow bends, your intensity level goes up, and your breath will get tighter. You will be able to manipulate your feet much easier, but it comes at a cost: you're more or less holding your breath. In this week, you'll learn how to regulate between easy breath with straight arms, and restricted breath with bent arms.

WEEK 4	
Monday	Rest day
Tuesday	Explore elbow-breath relationship
	• Warm-up
	• Hangboard
	• Three block exercises
	• IYTs
Wednesday	Fitness day
Thursday	Project boulder problems
	• Warm-up
	• Project
	• Wrist routine
Friday	Rest day
Weekend	Climb for Fun Day
	• Warm-up

Monday
Rest day.

Tuesday
Understand the relationship between elbow and breath on the hangboard. The program:

▶ Warm-up (page 198)

▶ Hangboard: Seven on/three off

• Pick an edge that gets you pumped after three sets

- Do seven-second hangs with a three-second rest between each, using three arm positions:
    - 90-degree bend in the elbow
    - 120-degree bend in the elbow
    - 170-degree bend in the elbow
- Four-minute rest between sets
- 2–5 sets

▶ These three exercises* are done in a block, which makes a single set.

- Pinch pull-ups (3–5); rest 30 seconds
- Negative push-ups (60 seconds); rest 30 seconds
- Negative pull-ups (60 seconds; page 205)
- Rest three minutes and repeat for 2–4 sets

The goal is not to complete the full minute. The goal is to stay aware and correct course when your form or quality drops. Being tired is OK, but lazy behavior is not OK.

▶ IYTs

- 0–5 pounds
- Fifteen reps
- 3-minute rest between sets
- 2–4 sets

Hangboard: Seven On / Three Off

This is great for understanding the relationship between the elbow and the breath. Do the first seven seconds on with a nice, clean lockoff. Dig deep—your core, your focus, your eyes will be stern. Then take three seconds off to soften and catch your breath. For the next seven, have a nice slight bend in the elbow, but keep the same hard focus and intensity. Then come down. The last seven seconds, do more of a straight-arm deadhang with shoulders and fingers engaged.

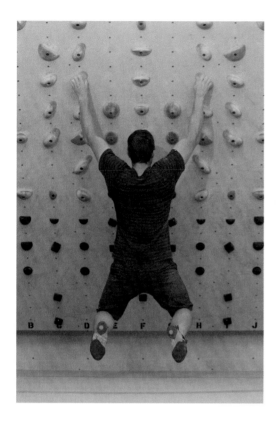 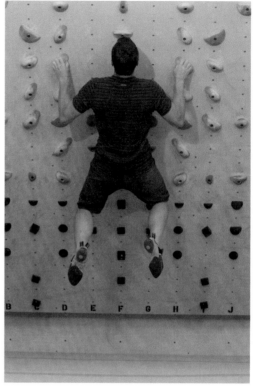

Pinch Pull-Ups

A system board is ideal, but you can use a hangboard, too. Find something that's shoulder-width, just like a pull-up. Pinching requires using your thumb for full-hand engagement. Squeeze and pull, aiming to do two to five pull-ups. If you have to put a foot on a box or step to complete these, do it.

Negative Push-Ups

Similar to negative pull-ups, this is just like a normal push-up with a slower down count. Push all the way up to the top of the push-up, then lower on a three- to five-second count. Quickly spike back up. Watch out for the lower back sag; keep a firm plank position. When you get tired, you might need to drop to your knees.

Wednesday

Fitness day. The program:

▶ Cardio (30 minutes)

▶ These six exercises* are done in a block, which makes a single set.

- Push-ups (60 seconds); rest 30 seconds

- Leg lifts (60 seconds); rest 30 seconds

- Right-side plank (60 seconds); rest 30 seconds

- Left-side plank (60 seconds); rest 30 seconds

- V-ups (60 seconds); rest 30 seconds

- Air squats (60 seconds)

- Rest three minutes and repeat for 2–4 sets

The goal is not to complete the full minute. The goal is to stay aware and correct course when your form or quality drops. Being tired is OK, but lazy behavior is not OK.

▶ Band exercises (page 200)

- Easy band

- Three exercises; no rest between exercises

- Fifteen reps each

- 3-minute rest between sets

- 2–4 sets

Thursday

Projecting boulder problems. The program:

▶ Warm-up

▶ Project

- Pick a climb you can send in two to three attempts

- Make one to four attempts (that's one set)

- Take a 10- to 20-minute rest between sets

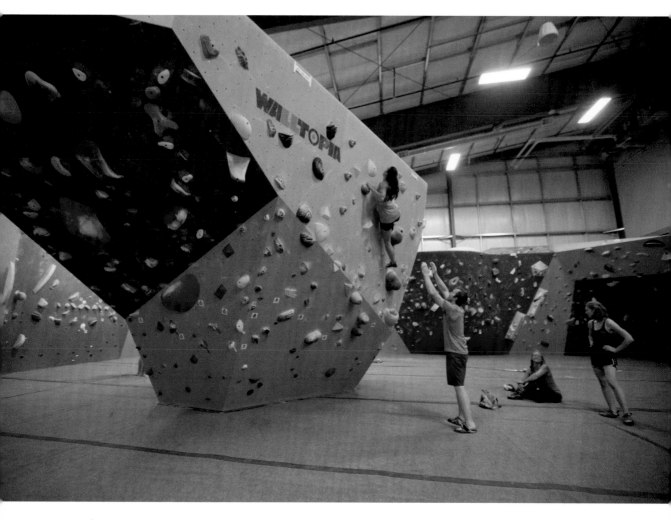

▶ Wrist routine

- Light weight

- Four exercises; no rest between exercises

- Fifteen reps each

- 3-minute rest between sets

- 2–4 sets

Bouldering Project Day

Today is about trying hard, not sending. Learn to grab small holds and move your body in an athletic way. Choose problems where you are able to complete two-thirds of the climb in three attempts. If you're doing it in one to two tries, the problems are too easy. If you recall your Top 6 Problems average, these projects might be just one step higher than your single best grade. Remember that when you try hard, you'll naturally get tense. You experience those moments when you get a better hold—remember that "good" is relative; learn to relax. Regain your breath. Recalibrate your eyes.

Friday

Rest day.

Weekend

Climb for fun at least one day, or two if you'd like, or do another moderate activity for one day, such as a hike or a bike ride.

WEEK 5: REST AND RECOVER

This week emphasizes the importance of rest. The schedule is more laid-back to give your body a chance to recover. An option if you're really trashed: Take this week off. You've been working hard weeks two, three, and four. You deserve this. If your body is feeling tweaky or tired, take time completely off. You may not even

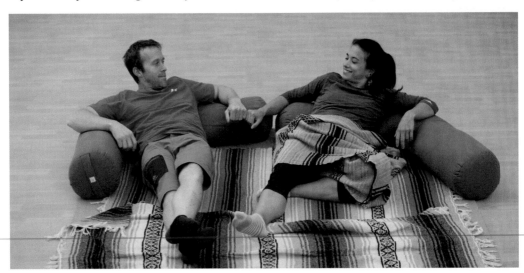

want to climb this week. You might just come into the gym and do a little bit of cardio or fitness. Rest is when your body gets stronger. Take care of yourself this week because in the next few weeks, you will dig deeper and push harder than you have so far.

WEEK 5	
Monday	Rest day
Tuesday	Rest and recover day
	• Warm-up
	• Free climb (sport or bouldering)
	• IYTs
Wednesday	Fitness day
Thursday	Rest and recover day
	• Warm-up
	• Free climb (sport or bouldering)
	• Wrist routine
Friday	Rest day
Weekend	Climb for Fun Day
	• Warm-up

Monday

Rest day.

Tuesday

Rest and recover. The program:

▶ Warm-up (page 198)

▶ Free day (sport climbing or bouldering)

▶ IYTs (page 206)

  • 0–5 pounds

  • Fifteen reps

  • 3-minute rest between sets

  • 2–4 sets

Free day!

Climb or boulder for fun for an hour or so. Call up those friends you've been ignoring because you've been training so hard.

Wednesday

Rest and recover. The program:

- ▶ Cardio (20 minutes)
- ▶ Band exercises (page 200)
  - Easy band
  - Three exercises; no rest between exercises
  - Fifteen reps each
  - 3-minute rest between sets
  - 2–4 sets

Thursday

Rest and recover. The program:

- ▶ Warm-up (page 198)
- ▶ Free day (bouldering focus)
- ▶ Wrist routine (page 201)
  - Light weight
  - Four exercises; no rest between exercises
  - Fifteen reps each
  - 3-minute rest between sets
  - 2–4 sets

Friday

Rest day.

Weekend

Climb for fun at least one day, or two if you'd like, or do another moderate activity for one day, such as a hike or a bike ride.

WEEK 6: INCREASING INTENSITY

Back to work! Week 6 is similar to Week 4, but we'll refine your intensity level. Build on the concept of contrast, so easy climbing is really easy and restful. Then, when it gets hard, meet the challenge by revving that engine. Work on your fingers through hangboarding and projecting boulders. When you're working fitness and resting between cycles, really breathe it out—though right before you start that next set, your brow should change; your breath should change. Same thing goes for working your projects.

WEEK 6	
Monday	Rest day
Tuesday	Express high/low intensity
	• Warm-up
	• Hangboard
	• Three block exercises
	• IYTs
Wednesday	Fitness day
Thursday	Project boulders with high/low intensity
	• Warm-up
	• Bouldering project
	• Wrist routine
Friday	Rest day
Weekend	Climb for Fun Day
	• Warm-up

Monday

Rest day.

Tuesday

Express intensity in the highs and lows. The program:

▶ Warm-up (page 198)

▶ Hangboard: Seven on/three off (page 218)

- Pick an edge that gets you pumped after four sets.

- Do seven-second hangs with three-second rests between each, using three arm positions:

    - 90-degree bend in the elbow

    - 120-degree bend in the elbow

    - 170-degree bend in the elbow

- four-minute rest between sets

- 2–5 sets

▶ These three exercises* are done in a block, which makes a single set.

- Pinch pull-ups (3–5; rest 30 seconds) (page 219)

- Negative push-ups (60 seconds; rest 30 seconds) (page 219)

- Negative pull-ups (60 seconds) (page 205)

- Rest three minutes and repeat for 2–4 sets

The goal is not to complete the full minute. The goal is to stay aware and correct course when your form or quality drops. Being tired is OK, but lazy behavior is not OK.

▶ IYTs (page 206)

- 0–5 pounds

- Fifteen reps

- 3-minute rests between sets

- 2–4 sets

Wednesday

Fitness day, but still express intensity through highs and lows. The program:

▶ Cardio (30 minutes)

▶ These six exercises* are done in a block, which makes a single set.

- Push-ups (60 seconds); rest 30 seconds (page 208)

- Leg lifts (60 seconds); rest 30 seconds (page 208)

- Right-side plank (60 seconds); rest 30 seconds (page 208)

- Left-side plank (60 seconds); rest 30 seconds (page 208)

- V-ups (60 seconds); rest 30 seconds (page 214)

- Squat jumps (60 seconds)

- Rest 3 minutes and repeat for 2–4 sets

The goal is not to complete the full minute. The goal is to stay aware and correct course when your form or quality drops. Being tired is OK, but lazy behavior is not OK.

▶ Band exercises (page 200)

- Easy band

- Three exercises, no rest between exercises

- Fifteen reps each

- 3-minute rest between sets

- 2–4 sets

Squat Jumps

Climbing is all about those legs, and this builds foundational strength a step beyond the traditional air squat. Start with your feet shoulder-width apart, with your weight distributed on your heels. Squat down. Your arms might move a little bit more than in an air squat because you are generating a lot more power. Drop down, explode

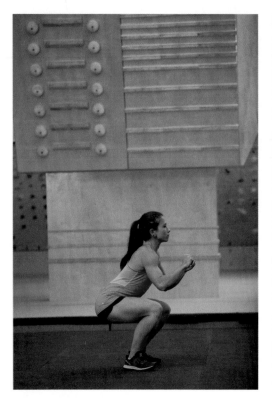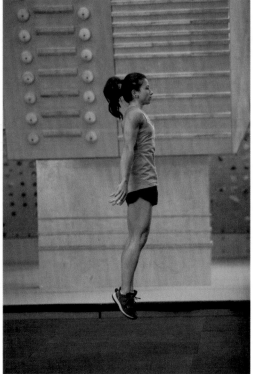

up through your legs, drive through your toes, jump into the air, and, when you come back down, gently drop right back down into another air squat. Then explode back up.

Thursday

Project boulders with high intensity when climbing and low intensity when resting. The program:

▶ Warm-up (page 198)

▶ Bouldering: Project day (page 222)

- Pick a climb you can send in two to four attempts

- Make one to four attempts (that's one set)

- Take an eight- to fifteen-minute rest between sets

- Repeat this cycle for one to three different climbs

▶ Wrist routine (page 201)

- Light weight

- Four exercises; no rest between exercises

- Fifteen reps each

- 3-minute rests between sets

- 2–4 sets

Friday

Rest day.

Weekend

Climb for fun at least one day, or two if you'd like, or do another moderate activity for one day, such as a hike or a bike ride.

WEEK 7: TRYING YOUR HARDEST

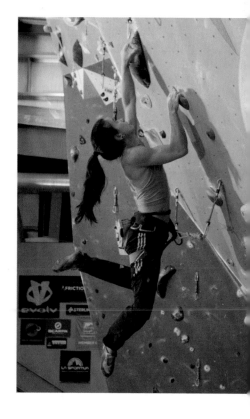

Become a machine. This week, you're going to get exhausted and then have to put on your game face and climb. Your goal: Be a warrior going into battle without fearing death. This week is all about training your performance. You will suffer in fitness, then immediately go and do some climbing. You will feel all slouchy and tired. But correct your posture, hold eye contact, and be focused. You won't send every climb; the intent isn't even to finish the climbs. You should fall near the top, because that means you could not push any farther, you could not dig any deeper. When you touch the ground again, either after bouldering or on a rope, you should look back and think, "Yeah, that was awesome. There was nothing more I could do."

WEEK 7	
Monday	Rest day
Tuesday	Find Your Performance Face
	• Warm-up
	• Fitness super sets
	• IYTs
Wednesday	Fitness day
Thursday	Find Your Performance Face with Difficult Climbing
	• Warm-up
	• 4x4 with fitness
	• Wrist routine
Friday	Rest Day
Weekend	Climb for Fun Day
	• Warm-up

Monday

Rest day.

Tuesday

Find your performance face. The program:

▶ Warm-up (page 198)

▶ Super sets with fitness: Do these four exercises,* then do your chosen route three times in a row, or do five-minute boulders for a bouldering set. This is one set.

- Push-ups (60 seconds); rest 30 seconds (page 208)

- Jumping pull-ups (60 seconds); rest 30 seconds (page 216)

- Box jumps (60 seconds); rest 30 seconds

- Planks (60 seconds)

- Rest three minutes; then repeat the whole set three times (four sets total), climbing a different route for each set. Anticipate how tired you'll feel, and adjust your approach as necessary.

The goal is not to complete the full minute. The goal is to stay aware and correct course when your form or quality drops. Being tired is OK, but lazy behavior is not OK.

▶ IYTs (page 206)

- 0–5 pounds
- Fifteen reps
- Three-minute rests between sets
- 2–4 sets

Box Jumps

You need to choose an appropriately sized box—one you can jump on, but that might make you hesitate when you get tired. Stand like you would for an air squat, squat down, then explode up onto the box. When you hit the top of the box, stand up and correct your spine, standing tall and proud. When you get tired, you will slouch and your heels might not get on the box. When this happens, take the time to compose yourself and repeat the motion with full force.

Planks

Planks are about feeling where your core is, or where your hips are, in relation to the rest of your body. Go onto your forearms with elbows under your shoulders, your back straight, and your hips in line with your toes and shoulders. If your shoulders get too tired, go from your forearms up to your hands to do a full plank.

Super Sets with Fitness

In a super set, you will get sufficiently tired in your gym's workout room, then choose a route to climb three times in succession, on toprope or lead. You will get very fatigued during this routine. Always double-check your harness and your tie-in point. Do three climbs. For the first climb you have a single goal: Climb from the bottom to the top. You should be able to complete it. For climbs two and three (they can be different or the same), complete three-quarters of the climb and hopefully fall in the top quarter. Push yourself to that absolute limit. You want to know how deep you can dig. Try your absolute hardest.

Focused on bouldering? Do five-minute boulders instead.

▶ Pick a problem at or just below your onsight level. Climb this two to four times in five minutes.

▶ After a 30-second break, do one minute of push-ups.

▶ After a 30-second break, do one minute of jumping pull-ups.

▶ After a 30-second break, do one minute of box jumps.

▶ After a 30-second break, do one minute of planks.

▶ That is a single set. Repeat for 2–4 sets.

Wednesday

Fitness day. The program:

▶ Cardio (30 minutes)

▶ These five exercises* are done in a block, which makes it a single set.

- Burpees (60 seconds); rest 30 seconds

- Leg lifts (60 seconds); rest 30 seconds (page 208)

- Planks (60 seconds); rest 30 seconds

- V-ups (60 seconds); rest 30 seconds (page 214)

- Squat jumps (60 seconds) (page 227)

- Rest three minutes and repeat for 2–4 sets

The goal is not to complete the full minute. The goal is to stay aware and correct course when your form or quality drops. Being tired is OK, but lazy behavior is not OK.

▶ Band exercises (page 200)

- Easy band

- Three exercises; no rest between exercises

- Fifteen reps each

- 3-minute rests between sets

- 2–4 sets

Burpees

These build core strength and explosive power through one difficult motion. Start standing, then drive and jump up, throwing your hands above your head. When

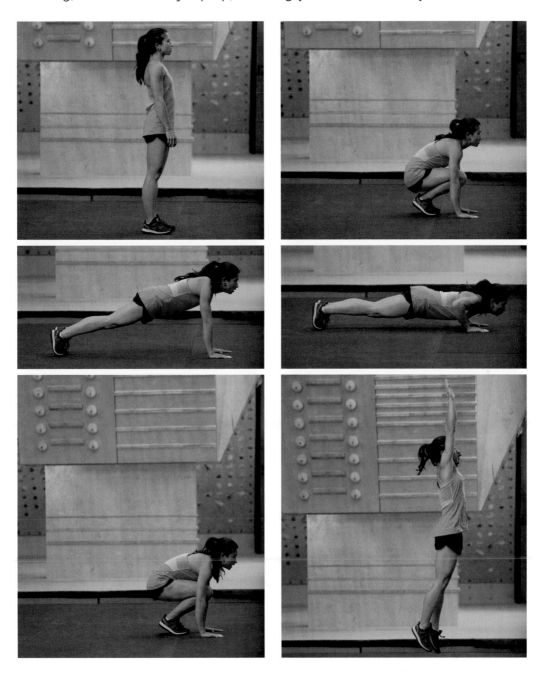

you come back down, drop down into a push-up position and lower your body all the way to the ground. Push up and jump your feet to your hands, and in one fluid motion jump up again, hands over your head. Repeat.

Thursday

Find your performance face with difficult climbing plus fitness. The program:

▶ Warm-up (page 198)

▶ 4x4 with fitness: Do these four exercises,* then do your four chosen boulder problems, making sure to complete the climbing portion in less than 20 minutes. This is one set.

- Push-ups (60 seconds; rest 30 seconds) (page 208)

- Jumping pull-ups (60 seconds; rest 30 seconds) (page 216)

- Box jumps (60 seconds; rest 30 seconds) (page 231)

- Planks (60 seconds) (page 231)

- Rest three minutes; then repeat three times (four sets total), climbing the same four boulder problems every time. Anticipate how tired you'll feel and adjust your approach as necessary.

The goal is not to complete the full minute. The goal is to stay aware and correct course when your form or quality drops. Being tired is OK, but lazy behavior is not OK.

▶ Wrist routine (page 201)

- Light weight

- Four exercises; no rest between exercises

- Fifteen reps each

- 3-minute rests between sets

- 2–4 sets

4x4 with Fitness

This is about suffering. Get tired in the fitness area, then head to the bouldering area with four problems in mind. The first should be easy and confidence-building.

The second and third should be challenging and physically sustained. The fourth should be at your limit. You get three attempts per problem, and your goal is to complete the four problems within twenty minutes. If you don't finish a particular problem in three gos, do not give it a fourth go. Once you complete these four problems, that is called a 1x4. Now get back into the fitness room and repeat the exercises and climbing until you've completed the 4x4. If you're finishing the boulder problems in less than twelve minutes, they're too easy. If you finish in thirteen minutes or longer, then rest the remaining time until it's been twenty minutes.

Friday
Rest day.

Weekend
Climb for fun at least one day, or two if you'd like, or do another moderate activity for one day, such as a hike or a bike ride.

WEEK 8: MATCH MENTAL GAME WITH PERFORMANCE

This week offers up another dose of performance training. Anticipate when you need to correct course and focus on what you want to happen. It's not about perfection but about becoming a better version of you.

We will now start building on anticipation. Before you go into the fitness room, before you begin to suffer, anticipate your behaviors. You shouldn't have to correct course from being slouchy and tired to warrior mode, because you've already anticipated that behavior and prevented it completely. Learn to understand yourself.

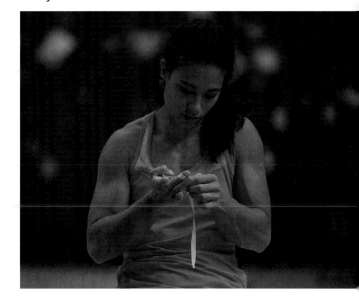

WEEK 8		
Monday	Rest day	
Tuesday	Correct Anticipated Behaviors	
	• Warm-up	
	• Super fitness sets	
	• IYTs	
Wednesday	Fitness day	
Thursday	4x4 with Fitness	
	• Warm-up	
	• 4x4 with fitness	
	• Wrist routine	
Friday	Rest Day	
Weekend	Climb for Fun Day	
	• Warm-up	

Monday
Rest day.

Tuesday
Anticipate your behavior and correct direction before it happens. The program:

▶ Warm-up (page 198)

▶ Super sets with fitness (page 231): Do these four exercises,* then do your chosen route three times in a row, or do five-minute boulders for a bouldering focus. This is one set.

- Push-ups (60 seconds); rest 30 seconds (page 208)

- Jumping pull-ups (60 seconds); rest 30 seconds (page 216)

- Box jumps (60 seconds); rest 30 seconds (page 231)

- Planks (60 seconds) (page 231)

- Rest three minutes; then repeat three times (four sets total), climbing a different route for each set. Anticipate how tired you'll feel and adjust your approach as necessary.

The goal is not to complete the full minute. The goal is to stay aware and correct course when your form or quality drops. Being tired is OK, but lazy behavior is not OK.

▶ IYTs (page 206)

- 0–5 pounds

- Fifteen reps

- 3-minute rests between sets

- 2–4 sets

Wednesday

Fitness day, while avoiding the tired slouch before it happens. The program:

▶ Cardio (30 minutes)

▶ These five exercises* are done in a block, which makes a single set.

- Burpees (60 seconds; rest 30 seconds) (page 233)

- Leg lifts (60 seconds; rest 30 seconds) (page 208)

- Planks (60 seconds; rest 30 seconds) (page 231)

- V-ups (60 seconds; rest 30 seconds) (page 214)

- Squat jumps (60 seconds) (page 227)

- Rest three minutes and repeat for 2–4 sets

The goal is not to complete the full minute. The goal is to stay aware and correct course when your form or quality drops. Being tired is OK, but lazy behavior is not OK.

▶ Band exercises (page 200)

- Easy band

- Three exercises; no rest between exercises

- Fifteen reps each

- 3-minute rests between sets

- 2–4 sets

Thursday
4x4 with fitness; anticipate your behavior and change course for the positive. The program:

▶ Warm-up (page 198)

▶ 4x4 with fitness (page 234): Do these four exercises,* then do your four chosen boulder problems, making sure to complete the climbing portion in less than twenty minutes. This is one set.

- Push-ups (60 seconds; rest 30 seconds) (page 208)

- Jumping pull-ups (60 seconds; rest 30 seconds) (page 216)

- Box jumps (60 seconds; rest 30 seconds) (page 231)

- Planks (60 seconds) (page 231)

- Rest three minutes; then repeat three times (four sets total), climbing the same four boulder problems every time. Anticipate how tired you'll feel and adjust your approach as necessary.

The goal is not to complete the full minute. The goal is to stay aware and correct course when your form or quality drops. Being tired is OK, but lazy behavior is not OK.

▶ Wrist routine (page 201)

- Light weight

- Four exercises; no rest between exercises

- Fifteen reps each

- 3-minute rests between sets

- 2–4 sets

Friday
Rest day.

Weekend
Climb for fun at least one day, or two if you'd like, or do another moderate activity for one day, such as a hike or a bike ride.

WEEK 9: REACHING PEAK PERFORMANCE

You've done all your training and suffering. Now it's preparing for glory. Week 9 is about tapering and learning what your new body—your upgraded machine—is all about. You're either resting or performing. Resting means totally chilling, letting your body recover. Performing means learning how to put on the best show, the best performance. Your efforts should inspire others to push their energy to you, to cheer you on. Seek that kind of response from your peers. Learn how to put on a good show.

WEEK 9	
Monday	Rest day
Tuesday	See How Far You've Come
	Warm-up
	Top 4 Routes / Top 6 Problems
Wednesday	Fitness day
Thursday	See How Far You've Come
	Warm-up
	Bouldering Top 6 Problems
Friday	Rest day
Weekend	Climb for Fun Day
	Warm-up

Monday

Rest day.

Tuesday

Get a snapshot of how far you've come with your Top 4 Routes or Top 6 Problems. Today's work:

▶ Warm-up (page 198)

▶ Top 4 Routes* (page 199)

If you are focused on bouldering, you'll do your Top 6 Problems instead.

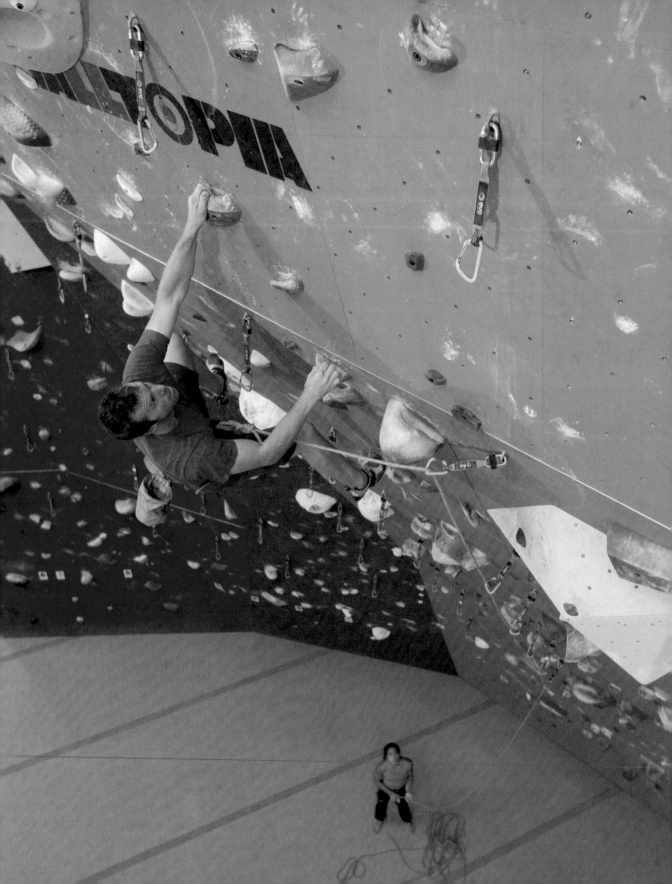

Wednesday

Relax, getting to know the new machine that is your body.

▶ Cardio (30 minutes—that's it!)

Thursday

Getting a snapshot of how far you've come with your Top 6 Problems. Today's work:

▶ Warm-up (page 198)

▶ Bouldering Top 6 (page 202)

Friday

Rest day.

Weekend

Climb for fun at least one day, or two if you'd like, or do another moderate activity for one day, such as a hike or a bike ride.

WEEK 10: USE YOUR NEWFOUND FITNESS!

Remember your Week 1 goals, and go send. That's why you wrote them down—so it's not some vague thing in your head. It doesn't always click right away. Be patient. Sometimes people have already seen improvements. Sometimes it takes a while to connect. There is no right or wrong. It's about what happens to you; it's your journey. You need to rest and perform. Take a few weeks before you start training seriously again. Enjoy your new strengths by climbing hard, trying things above your level, falling, and learning on each route or problem. Believe in yourself, and take the time and energy to enjoy what you're doing right now.

INDEX OF EXERCISES: QUICK REFERENCE

We've all been there: You want to go to the gym to get a great workout, but you don't quite know what to do. Maybe you only have an hour and want to get completely thrashed, or maybe you just want to move around a bit and focus on fun. Whatever your situation—time, psych level, commitment, partner availability—and whatever you want to improve upon, there's a workout in here for you. Below is a quick reference guide to the exercises in this book, sorted by how and what you want to train.

What Do You Want to Train?		
Strength: Full Body	Bouldering Intervals	Page 36
	World Cup Simulator	Page 44
	Tales of Power	Page 49
	4x4s	Page 53
	Circuits	Page 53
	Treadwall	Page 74
	Strong Circuits	Page 167
	Home Improvement	Page 171
	Freaky Fit	Page 177
	Essential Yoga	Page 179
	Shoulders and Hips Strengthening	Page 191
Strength: Fingers/Forearms	Hangboarding 101	Page 100
	Hangboard Repeaters	Page 103
	Fingerboard Moving Hangs	Page 117
	Hangboard Ladders	Page 128
	Digit Dialing	Page 131
	Lockoffs	Page 43
Strength: Core	Peter Pans	Page 43
	Complete Core	Page 142
	Suspended Circuits	Page 157

Strength: Upper Body	Project, Push-Up, Pull-Up	Page 37
	Upper Body Tabata	Page 156
	6-Second Death Drop	Page 111
	Perfect Pull-Ups	Page 112
Strength: Legs	Do the Legwork	Page 152
Strength: Shoulders	Make Big Moves on the Campus Board	Page 108
	Ladders on the Bachar Ladder	Page 119
Strength: Injury Prevention	Targeted Opposition	Page 120
	Shoulder Routine	Page 123
	Wrist Routine	Page 124, 201
	Protect Elbows and Shoulders	Page 124
Technique	Drills	Page 39
	Create a Crux	Page 50
	MoonBoard	Page 56
	Bookends	Page 38
	Flash Sessions	Page 47
	Limit Bouldering	Page 55
	Traverse Eliminates	Page 82
	Climb with Grace on the System Board	Page 106
Endurance	Climb Forever Arc Sets	Page 70
	Leapfrog	Page 73
	Pyramids	Page 77
	Roped Intervals	Page 78
	Volume for Points	Page 80
	Laps	Page 81
	3x10 Intervals	Page 84
	Up-Downs	Page 86

On a Time Crunch?		
Less than 1 Hour	Make Any Exercise More Climbing Specific	Page 137
	Traverse Eliminates	Page 82
	Hangboarding 101	Page 100
	Hangboard Repeaters	Page 103

	Climb with Grace on the System Board	Page 106
	Make Big Moves on the Campus Board	Page 108
	6-Second Death Drop	Page 111
	Perfect Pull-Ups	Page 112
	Fingerboard Moving Hangs	Page 117
	Ladders on the Bachar Ladder	Page 119
	Targeted Opposition	Page 120
	Shoulder Routine	Page 123
	Wrist Routine	Page 124, 201
	Protect Elbows and Shoulders	Page 124
	Hangboard Ladders	Page 128
	Digit Dialing	Page 131
	Complete Core	Page 142
	Do the Legwork	Page 152
	Upper Body Tabata	Page 156
	Suspended Circuits	Page 157
	Strong Circuits	Page 167
	Home Improvement	Page 171
	Freaky Fit	Page 177
	Essential Yoga	Page 179
1–2 Hours	Lockoffs	Page 43
	Peter Pans	Page 43
	Flash Sessions	Page 47
	Tales of Power	Page 49
	Limit Bouldering	Page 55
	Leapfrog	Page 73
	Roped Intervals	Page 78
	Up-Downs	Page 86
	Shoulders and Hips Strengthening	Page 191
3+ Hours	Project, Push-Up, Pull-Up	Page 37
	World Cup Simulator	Page 44
	4x4s	Page 53
	Circuits	Page 53
	Climb Forever Arc Sets	Page 70

	Pyramids	Page 77
	Laps	Page 81
	3x10 Intervals	Page 84
Customizable Time	Bouldering Intervals	Page 36
	Bookends	Page 38
	Create a Crux	Page 50
	MoonBoard	Page 56
	Treadwall	Page 74
	Volume for Points	Page 80

Got a Buddy?

With a Partner	Boulder Intervals	Page 36
	Leapfrog	Page 73
	3x10 Intervals	Page 84
	Ladders on the Bachar Ladder	Page 119
Going Solo	Project, Push-Up, Pull-Up	Page 37
	Bookends	Page 38
	Lockoffs	Page 43
	World Cup Simulator	Page 44
	Flash Sessions	Page 47
	Tales of Power	Page 49
	4x4s	Page 53
	Circuits	Page 53
	Limit Bouldering	Page 55
	Treadwall	Page 74
	Traverse Eliminates	Page 82
	Hangboarding 101	Page 100
	Hangboard Repeaters	Page 103
	Make Big Moves on the Campus Board	Page 108
	6-Second Death Drop	Page 111
	Perfect Pull-Ups	Page 112
	Fingerboard Moving Hangs	Page 117
	Targeted Opposition	Page 120
	Shoulder Routine	Page 123

	Wrist Routine	Page 124, 201
	Protect Elbows and Shoulders	Page 124
	Hangboard Ladders	Page 128
	Digit Dialing	Page 131
	Make Any Exercise More Climbing Specific	Page 137
	Complete Core	Page 142
	Do the Legwork	Page 152
	Upper Body Tabata	Page 156
	Suspended Circuits	Page 157
	Strong Circuits	Page 167
	Home Improvement	Page 171
	Freaky Fit	Page 177
	Essential Yoga	Page 179
	Shoulders and Hips Strengthening	Page 191
With or Without Partner	Peter Pans	Page 43
	Create a Crux	Page 50
	MoonBoard	Page 56
	Climb Forever Arc Sets	Page 70
	Pyramids	Page 77
	Roped Intervals	Page 78
	Volume for Points	Page 80
	Laps	Page 81
	Up-Downs	Page 86
	Climb with Grace on the System Board	Page 106

Exercise Intensity		
High Intensity	Project, Push-Up, Pull-Up	Page 37
	Peter Pans	Page 43
	World Cup Simulator	Page 44
	4x4s	Page 53
	Circuits	Page 53
	Climb Forever Arc Sets	Page 70
	Traverse Eliminates	Page 82

	Make Big Moves on the Campus Board	Page 108
	Upper Body Tabata	Page 156
	Suspended Circuits	Page 157
	Strong Circuits	Page 167
	Home Improvement	Page 171
	Shoulders and Hips	Page XXX
Moderate Intensity	Bouldering Intervals	Page 36
	Flash Sessions	Page 47
	Tales of Power	Page 49
	Create a Crux	Page 50
	Limit Bouldering	Page 55
	MoonBoard	Page 56
	Leapfrog	Page 73
	Pyramids	Page 77
	Roped Intervals	Page 78
	Volume for Points	Page 80
	3x10 Intervals	Page 84
	Up-Downs	Page 86
	Hangboarding 101	Page 100
	Hangboard Repeaters	Page 103
	Climb with Grace on the System Board	Page 106
	Perfect Pull-Ups	Page 112
	Fingerboard Moving Hangs	Page 117
	Ladders on the Bachar Ladder	Page 119
	Digit Dialing	Page 131
	Complete Core	Page 142
	Do the Legwork	Page 152
	Freaky Fit	Page 177
Low Intensity	Bookends	Page 38
	Laps	Page 81
	Treadwall	Page 74
	6-Second Death Drop	Page 111
	Targeted Opposition	Page 120
	Shoulder Routine	Page 123

	Wrist Routine	Page 124, 201
	Protect Elbows and Shoulders	Page 124
	Hangboard Ladders	Page 128
	Make Any Exercise More Climbing Specific	Page 137
	Essential Yoga	Page 179

Let's Talk Long-Term Goals . . .		
I Need a Program	Boulder Three Grades Harder	Page 61
	Get Strong for Steep Sport	Page 87
	Climb 5.12	Page 94
	Climb a Grade Harder	Page 195

GLOSSARY OF TERMS

ANCHOR: The fixed equipment at the top of a route where a toprope is attached, or where the rope can be clipped for safe lowering when lead climbing.

APE INDEX: The length of a person's wingspan, from fingertip to fingertip, which can impact a climber's ability to reach a hold. Often an ape index is about the same as a person's height, but if it's more or less, it's referred to "positive" or "negative." A person who is 5'6" tall and has a 5'8" ape index would have a "plus 2" ape index.

ARETE: An outward-facing corner feature, like the edge of a building where two planes meet.

AUTOBELAY: A device that hangs at the top of the wall and provides toprope protection for roped climbers without the need for a partner.

BACHAR LADDER: A training tool in which the goal is to campus between large plastic tubes on a hanging ladder that angles diagonally upward.

BACK-STEP: A movement in which the outside of one hip is turned into the wall, and the foot on that same side steps up on a hold beneath the hip, with the outside edge of the foot on the foothold.

BARNDOOR: Any move in climbing that results in one side of the body swinging out away from the wall, like a barn door opening on its hinges.

BELAY: The protection for a roped climber when he or she falls, which is provided by a partner (the belayer) who secures the rope with specialized equipment (belay device).

BETA: Information on how to complete a climb, including specific moves, rests, and hold types.

BICYCLE: Foot movement that involves using both feet on the same hold. One foot pushes on the front of the hold with the bottom of the toes while the other pulls against the back of the hold with the top of the toes.

BOLT: A metal expansion bolt used as a protection point for sport or lead climbing.

BOULDERING: A type of climbing done without a rope on standalone boulders or short cliff lines, where the climber ventures 15 to 20 feet off the ground. During a fall, a climber lands on a soft, foam pad (crash pad).

BUMP: A move in which you use a specific hold just for a split second before moving to another, usually better, hold.

BURN: Each try on a problem or route.

CAMPUS: To climb without using your feet, meaning they hang in the air while you surge between handholds.

CAMPUS BOARD: A series of wooden rungs of varying shapes and sizes that are set a specific distance apart, with the goal of climbing/surging between them without using your feet. This training tool helps build power.

CHALK BAG: A small bag attached to your waist that holds chalk for keeping your hands dry.

CHALK POT: A bag, usually larger than a chalk bag, that holds chalk but does not attach to your body, and instead sits on the floor. Used specifically for bouldering.

CLEAN: To climb something cleanly is to climb it without falling or grabbing gear.

CORNER: An inward-facing corner feature, also referred to as a dihedral.

CRASH PAD: A soft foam pad used for fall protection while bouldering.

CRIMP: A small edge or lip that you can only get part of your fingertips on, necessitating closing your thumb against the index finger to use the grip.

CRUX: The hardest section or sequence on a climb.

DEADPOINT: A dynamic move in which one or both feet stay on the wall and you grab the target hold on the upward trajectory at the full extent of your reach.

DOWNCLIMB: To climb down a route or problem instead of up.

DROP-KNEE: A climbing technique in which the foot is placed out to the side on a hold, with the hip turned into the wall and the knee down and in, which torques the foot on the hold and extends your reach.

DYNAMIC: A climbing movement that uses momentum to reach holds.

DYNO: A dynamic move that involves jumping to reach a hold. Both feet leave the wall.

EDGE: A narrow ledgelike climbing hold. See also "crimp."

ELIMINATE: Climbing a route or boulder problem without using certain holds, in order to make it harder.

ELVIS LEG: Also referred to as sewing-machine leg, this occurs when you get nervous and/or fatigued on a climb and your leg and foot start shaking uncontrollably. Usually, the toe stays on the hold while the heel and ankle pump up and down as your quad and calf vibrate.

ENDURANCE: The ability to stay on the wall for a long period of time and to climb without getting tired and falling off.

FEATURE: A large aspect of the wall, like a corner, arête, roof, or slab.

FIGURE EIGHT: Also known as a figure eight follow-through, this is the knot that climbers commonly use to tie into the rope.

FINGER STRENGTH: This is a climber's ability to grip certain holds, and refers to a combination of muscle, tendon, ligament, and joint strength in the forearms, wrists, and hands.

FLAG: Any time you use your leg to maintain balance (instead of supporting weight), usually without that foot being on an actual hold.

FLAPPER: A skin injury in which a flap of skin is partially ripped off yet remains semi-attached. Often received in the beginning of a person's climbing career when the skin is soft and hasn't yet toughened up to withstand the rough texture of climbing holds.

FLASH: Successfully completing a climb the first time you try it, with prior knowledge of the moves and holds (perhaps provided by a friend). The first time you pull on to a climb is a "flash attempt."

FLASH-PUMP: When your forearms suddenly feel pumped, swollen, or tired on a climb, usually early in a climbing session when you're not properly warmed up.

GASTON: A type of sidepull gripped with the elbow out, palm toward the wall, and the thumb pointing downward.

GRADE: The number and letter rating given to a climb to denote difficulty. Some gyms use their own grading system (e.g., spots, colors), but typically boulder problems are graded on the V-scale (VB/V0 and up) and roped climbs on the Yosemite Decimal System (5.0 and up).

HANGBOARD: Also known as a fingerboard, this is a training tool with a specific set of holds on it. The climber hangs from holds for a certain amount of time, sometimes using added weight.

HEEL HOOK: By turning the knee out and placing the back of the heel on a hold, you can pull in with your leg to stay on the wall.

HOLD: These are what climbers use to move up a wall. In a gym, they're three-dimensional pieces of plastic attached to the climbing wall, and come in infinite shapes and sizes.

JIB: A super-small foothold.

JUG: Any climbing hold that is huge, incut, and easy to hang on to.

KNEEBAR: A climbing move in which you wedge your lower leg between two holds; the toes push against a foothold, which simultaneously presses your knee into another hold and takes some of the load off your arms.

LEAD CLIMBING: A type of roped climbing in which the climber moves up the wall and clips protection (bolts) as he or she goes. Lead climbing requires experienced and dialed-in systems.

LOCKOFF: A static move pulling down on one hold and keeping that engaged position while you reach up with the other arm.

MANTEL: Often done in bouldering, especially on a topout, this climbing press-up is the same idea as getting out of a swimming pool—you go from pulling on a hold to pushing down on it and bringing a foot up to rock over.

MATCH: This refers to putting both hands or both feet on one hold at the same time.

MAX EFFORT: This refers to a climbing move or weighted exercise that requires your hardest, or maximum, effort.

MONO: Any climbing hold where you can only use one finger; often refers to a mono pocket.

MOONBOARD: A small, standardized training wall built to certain specifications so you can climb the exact same problems as anyone else who has a MoonBoard.

NATURALS: In a climbing gym the walls can have bumps, divots, cracks, and edges built into the wall itself, instead of the bolt-on holds.

ONSIGHT: This is similar to a flash—successfully completing a climb the first time you try it—but involves not having any prior knowledge or beta about the climb.

OPEN FEET: On easy climbs, often routesetters will suggest "open feet," meaning you can use any footholds you want instead of sticking to certain ones.

OVERHANG: A section of wall that's steeper than vertical.

PINCH: A climbing hold that requires you to squeeze the hold between your thumb and other fingers.

PLATEAU: This refers to a period in your climbing when, despite training or climbing frequently, you're not seeing any noticeable improvement.

POCKET: A climbing hold that resembles a hole and only fits a certain number of fingers (e.g., a two-finger pocket).

POWER: High-intensity movement or maximum strength combined with speed; the explosive force recruited any time you use momentum. It's the ability to do a hard move quickly and forcefully. Climbers need this type of strength for dynamic moves.

POWER-ENDURANCE: The ability to sustain high-intensity movements, or being able to do many hard moves in a row. It's a combination of—you guessed it—power and endurance.

PROBLEM: The specific path taken by a climber when bouldering; a problem is what boulders call a specific climb.

PROJECT: A climb (roped or bouldering) that is at or above your limit, forcing you to try it over and over again (projecting), sometimes over the course of weeks or months before you succeed.

PUMPED: The forearm tiredness you get from climbing at your limit. The muscles feel swollen, making it hard to hold onto the wall.

QUICKDRAW: Also called a "draw," this nylon sling with a carabiner on either end is used to attach the rope to a bolt, or any other protection point.

REDPOINT: When you successfully climb a route without falling after having tried it repeatedly (projected).

ROOF: A steep overhang that's almost horizontal; a ceiling.

ROPED CLIMBING: Any type of climbing that involves a rope (e.g., lead climbing or toproping).

ROUTE: The specific path taken by a climber when roped climbing. A route is what a climb is called when roped climbing.

ROUTESETTING: Often shortened to "setting," this is the act of putting holds on the wall to create routes and problems. The people who do this at a gym are referred to as routesetters or setters, and depending on the gym, each "set" (or group of problems/routes) will be up anywhere from 4 weeks to a few months.

SANDBAG: When a climb is given a lower grade than its actual difficulty.

SCUM: Any time you use a part of your body that's not your fingers or your feet to adhere to the wall for balance or weight-bearing, like a hip scum or a head scum.

SEND: To complete a climb without falling.

SESSION: This refers to each time you go climb (e.g., "Monday's gym session was a lot better than Tuesday's).

SEQUENCE: The certain order of specific moves on a climb.

SIDEPULL: A type of hold you grab vertically, from either the left or the right side.

SIT-START: In bouldering, a problem that must be started by sitting on the ground.

SLAB: Any section of wall that's less than vertical.

SLACK: When roped climbing, this is the portion of the rope that's hanging loose. Sometimes the belayer needs to pull it in, and sometimes the belayer needs to give more slack so the climber can move freely or take a soft fall.

SLOPER: A rounded climbing hold with no positive edges to grab.

SMEAR: A foot move in which you use a large area of your forefoot, smeared or pasted on a hold or the wall itself—versus precisely placing the point of the big toe on a small section of a hold.

SPORT CLIMBING: A style of roped climbing in which the climber clips bolts for protection as he or she moves up the wall.

SPOTTING: When bouldering, this person helps guide a falling climber's body to a safe landing on the pads.

SPRAY: This has two meanings, both with negative connotations: offering unwanted beta to a fellow climber, and bragging (or talking a lot about) your own accomplishments.

STATIC: Doing climbing moves in a slow, controlled fashion—the opposite of a dynamic move.

STEEP: Any section of wall that's vertical or steeper.

STEM: Usually done in a corner or dihedral, where a climber has a foot on one face and the other foot on the other face in opposition.

STEP-THROUGH: A type of foot move in which one leg crosses the plane of the other leg to reach a foothold.

STICKY RUBBER: The specialized rubber found on climbing shoes that helps grip holds.

SYSTEM BOARD: A small climbing wall, sometimes a woody, in which the holds are mirrored on each side so you can perform the exact same movements on either side of your body. Often the wall is steep and the holds are small or sloping.

TAKE!: This is used as a command to your belayer when you want him or her to pull in all the slack in the rope and hold your weight, either to rest or after you've finished a climb and have clipped the anchor: "Jamie, take!"

TAPE: Some gyms use different-colored tape to denote which holds are part of a particular climb. Other gyms don't use tape and instead use hold colors for their routes.

TECHNIQUE: The way in which you move your body, legs, and arms as efficiently as possible, including footwork, body positioning, and sequencing.

TOE HOOK: This is a climbing move where, with your leg extended, you hook the top of your foot against a hold to stay on the wall.

TOEING IN: Using your toes to press down and pull in on a foothold to hold your hips into the wall, especially on overhangs.